I0697141

A
Perfect Family

Mary Joslyn

This book is a work of fiction. Names, characters, places, and incidents are the product of the author's imagination and are used fictitiously. Any resemblance to actual events, locales, or persons, living or dead, is coincidental.

All rights reserved. No part of this book may be used or reproduced in any manner whatsoever without express written permission, except in the case of brief quotations used in critical articles or reviews of this work.

A Perfect Family © 2023 by Mary Joslyn

Chapter 1

When Goldenrod was just eight years old, she told her mother, Helen that when she was grown, she would marry an architect, live in a log cabin in Canada and have eight children. And by the way, from then on, she would be called Denny. Not Goldenrod. Goldenrod was the name of an ugly common weed. Giving it to a child as a first name was just further evidence that fifteen-year-olds should not be having babies! "I was sixteen when you were born, dear. And I don't regret it one bit," Helen tweaked the proud little nose of her only daughter and mused the idea of her having eight children of her own someday. Denny promptly forgot the entire conversation, however, and buried herself in books. She forged new dreams of faraway places she would travel unhindered by any man or offspring. She modeled herself after Belle, from Beauty and the Beast collecting books wherever she could find them. Her mother's shelves were loaded with books on childbirth and anatomy containing strange pictures of nude laboring women with bulging nether parts covered in curly hair like beards extending across the inner thighs. It was alarming to explore her mother's midwifery textbooks and more than once she'd slammed the cover shut, revolted by what she saw. No, she didn't care for these illustrations and real photos. She wanted the written words. The more the better. She spent hours reading classics by Hemingway and Shakespeare. She devoured Little Women, A Tale of Two Cities, Pride and Prejudice.

She read all the books her aunt Rita gave her, authored by missionaries and Holocaust survivors like Elizabeth Elliot and Corrie Ten Boom, to spirit seeking Tom Brown and his wilderness walks, to Sidney Sheldon, Virginia Andrews, Danielle Steele, and Mary Higgins Clark, the last of which Denny agreed with her mother, were literary junk food. But her diet was insatiable, and she would read whatever she could get her hands on, eventually leading to studying journalism at Syracuse University, where she met Melissa.

Melissa Albrecht and Denny Kline were immediate friends. Some sweet pixie dust from heaven put them in the same dorm as roommates. They bonded over books, pursued the same degree, and once they confided in and got to know one another better, realized they had fatherlessness in common. Denny grew up in a house full of women; her mother Helen and her mother's two sisters, Aunt Diane and Aunt Rita. The three sisters were orphaned when Helen was just six. Rita was the oldest at 17, eleven years older than Helen, and Diane was in the middle at 13. At the time, Denny's aunt Rita took over the role of mom and did her best to care for her sisters. They managed to keep the farmhouse, and eventually Denny would be born outside under the sumac to a very young Helen. A teenage neighbor boy, Alex had fled at the prospect of fatherhood, joining the navy and leaving Helen and her older sisters to parent Denny. Helen was a young but loving mother, fiercely determined to do right by her little Goldenrod. She studied midwifery while her sisters helped care for Denny like she belonged to all three of them. The farmhouse was warm and full of life. Denny's childhood was rich and full, a boarding house bustling with activity; a revolving door of unwed teens who were pregnant or nursing babies, a cottage business of goat milk soaps, artisan breads. Warm days were filled with pulling weeds, milking goats, harvesting honey, and never-ending laundry on the clothesline. In the winter, it was quilt making and crocheting bags, sweaters, vests and mittens to sell at the indoor market. And spring was for tapping maple trees and cooking-down syrup. There was always plenty to do, and the women were thrifty and industrious so they could afford to continue on the farm and keep their land.

Melissa had been raised by the help. Her parents ignored her completely from birth, disappointed that she wasn't a boy, in the way one would snub a fish dinner being brought to the table when they had clearly ordered a steak. She was left in the home on a lakefront estate in Skaneateles with caretakers and nannies who were genuinely warm and attentive. But her parents were very busy delegates, thinking themselves important, traveling often, and expecting nothing of Melissa except that she not inconvenience them any more than she had already by being born. To fill the vast loneliness and the ache of rejection, Melissa disappeared into books. She was surrounded with rooms full of books and a library that was more grand than anything Denny had ever seen. She visited the Albrecht estate only once. And though she was in awe of the tall columns, the grand veranda, the manicured property and gardens, and most of all the library, she felt the vast emptiness of the place, and shuddered to think of her friend growing up in such rich splendor, cold as a refrigerator. It made Denny's heart ache for her. "From now on, you come to the farm on weekends," Denny told her firmly. "Bring all the belongings you want; We'll rent a U-Haul if we have to! But we're not staying here." Melissa didn't argue. Denny was like a warm blanket. Not only did they have favorite authors and stories in common, but Denny radiated love and confidence like Melissa had only dreamed of. She always wanted a schoolgirl friendship, but the wide hollow halls of her home only accommodated the dullest lecturers, mentors, and tutors. None of whom resembled the characters in her books; the tall smart Mr. Darcy, or the women clad in ruffles with bound waists, soft golden curls and alabaster skin. No one mysterious or interesting. Rather, the likes of Mister

Whipplan, a fat man in a bulging pinstriped vest with a bloated face and red blotchy patches on his skin and unruly gray tufts of hair coming from his ears and nostrils. He stood over her, the crumbs from his breakfast toast still lodged in his kinky beard moving with his every word. She tried to imagine him as a young man. Was it possible? Could he have ever been decent looking? She looked out the window so as not to stare at the crumbs as he talked and prayed to a God she had only heard of in books that someday she would have a bosom buddy. A true friend. A girl of her very own, to brush hair and play dolls and talk of boys while arranging blossoms of summer collected during stolen walks under a big blue sky that smiled down on them. This tiny dream was the only one she really had. And when Denny appeared like a jewel, hand-plucked out of the heavens and set twinkling perfectly right smack in the same little dorm room with Melissa Albrecht, she could hardly believe her luck. Denny was warm and wonderful. Whitty and brilliant. Her hair as blond as cornsilk glowing from the light that blazed within. There was nothing shallow or embellished about this beauty. All her light came from within and warmed everything from her crystal blue sapphire eyes to her warm golden hair, to her softly tanned skin. Melissa loved her immediately.

Denny was more guarded. Not for lack of trust as much as temperament. Denny did burn bright as a furnace on the inside, but she warmed up to others slowly and cautiously. She was independent and although she had a duty-to-serve quality about her in relation to everyone she met, she was in control of the how, when, and how much. Once she had accepted the responsibility of relationship, she was fiercely loyal, protective and consistent. Melissa became Denny's best friend and the recipient of any and all attentiveness aside from her studies.

Melissa Albrecht had big plans. She was driven in a way Denny never would be. She was restless, wound, studious, intense, determined. She worked and studied harder than anything Denny had seen. And she recruited all of Denny's free time to help with her latest venture. "I'll be damned if I'm waiting for some stupid piece of paper before I launch my magazine. I'll have a hundred thousand subscribers before my catwalk in cap and gown. And you'll be my chief editor," Melissa was never more focused in all her life. Now that she had someone in her corner, someone who cared for her, she began to believe what she always suspected. She wasn't a waste. She was somebody. She was strong, and able and impressive. She could do anything! Parents be damned. They never appreciated her. Appreciate? They never even acknowledged her. Well, she would not be sitting around a lonely castle ever again. She had things to do. And putting together a magazine was only the beginning.

When they finished at SU, they moved to New York City together. Melissa had achieved her goal and had a successful magazine off the ground even before they were seniors. But in a few short years, Denny returned to the farm. She had unwittingly been swept into her dear friend's frenzied life pace. Her trip home for her Aunt Diane's funeral extended longer and longer, an excuse she used to get away from the magazine and the city and to get some clarity. She hadn't realized how buried she was, and her mother helped Denny to ease the guilt of leaving Melissa with the workload. "You've always wanted to write, Denny. So take a little time off and rest. See what comes up." Her mom had a way of making life sound so easy-going. As if it would be absurd to plow ahead working if your heart is conflicted. Time must be taken, things weighed, observed. Let stillness come. And then see what unfolds. It amused Denny to think of the limitless energy Melissa had and how it had rubbed off on her. Yet with a little distance Denny realized it was more of a compulsion. She was not so much inspired as driven. Denny decided she wasn't doing Melissa any favors by helping her keep pace. They would both be dead by forty at the rate they were working. And so, Denny stayed. Her mother needed her. And she needed a break.

Chapter 2

In time, Melissa convinced Denny to return to New York for a visit. She invited Denny to a swanky party with a long list of interesting guests; a big-name restaurant critic known throughout New York's food scene, a renowned sculptor and painter, and a curator from the Metropolitan Museum of Art. Melissa tried to lure Denny with an architect from Canada, Max Belanger who partnered with his father Bishop Belanger, the Lloyd Wright of the Great White North. Denny had never heard of him, and she knew nothing of renowned architects. But Melissa persisted, reminding Denny that she would marry an architect and live in a log cabin in Canada with eight children.

"I was drunk," Denny said.

"Still, you said it."

"It's a silly story my mother tells. I don't even remember saying it." Denny sighed into the phone.

"Well, you remembered the story. Or else you wouldn't have spilled it in a drunk confession!"

Denny was aware of regarding only one thought concerning marriage. *Don't do it!* Apparently Melissa had different ideas for her. She had made a mental note of the buried wishes of her best friend, and when she heard about the guest list at this party, it clicked immediately. Besides, she was looking for an excuse to reconnect. Melissa was growing more and more concerned that she'd blown it, her best-ever friendship, by needing her too much. When Denny had not returned, the fear shook her terribly. She wasn't in the least upset that Denny had left her severely overworked and understaffed, Melissa was sure she'd pushed her too far. Denny didn't like the fast pace of a successful magazine. She wasn't crazy about the city. Melissa had kept her too busy for too long. And she had to make it up to her.

"Just come and stay with me. We'll catch a show, hit this party, and stay up all night catching up," Mel had whined. Denny's heart ached. She missed her terribly and could not refuse her. She left Croghan by bus to Utica and caught a train to Penn Station that Friday. Melissa picked her up brimming with enthusiasm and tight hugs. Denny knew they were in for a great weekend. Melissa was still running the magazine, and when Denny asked how it was going, Mel made a face with huge eyes and an overwhelmed expression. And then she frowned and looked intensely at Denny,

"You, my dear… should never have left! It's impossible without you," she heaved an exaggerated sigh and threw the back of her hand against her forehead with excessive drama. Then she gripped Denny by the shoulders looked her straight in the eyes and said, "It'll never be the same. Nothing will ever be right again," she pursed her lips and looked like she might cry. Denny saw a flash of deep loneliness, and knowing she wasn't exaggerating, pulled her in close and hugged her again, "I have missed you so," she squeezed her tight and kissed her on the cheek.

"Yes! But are you sorry you left?" Melissa carried on with the theatrics.

"No," she said quickly, but then seeing hurt in her eyes, "well, maybe a little. I do miss all the action around here. But I feel more sane back on the farm."

"Ah, screw sane," Mel laughed as she flagged a cab and they sped off to her flat chatting about all the plans for the weekend. Denny was surprised Melissa had completely cleared her schedule of work. There was a time when they worked together getting the magazine off the ground when Denny thought Melissa would never be able to keep such a maddening pace. But kept it she did. And she expected Denny to as well, working oblivious to the hours passing or life passing. Just buried under the next deadline, writing, editing, and always pressed for time. Melissa seemed unaffected. Rather, she thrived, requiring neither breaks, nor sleep. She devoured work as if it were a gourmet buffet and she was starving. The work itself was her reward. She required nothing else. Denny could meet obligations, but it wasn't with joy. She was burnt out. The job's unrelenting pace was a conveyor belt of endless and similar unfinished projects. Factory work where the shift doesn't end, the whistle never blows, and the work continues on even in sleep. Even the financial rewards, though generous, were not gratifying.

When she received the news from her mother, that her Aunt Diane had died, she came up for air for the first time in months, beckoned to the surface hearing her mother's voice from somewhere outside the thick smog of the city with its horns, sirens and constant barrage of noise. It was a call from another life. Had it been so long since she'd been home to the farm? When she arrived home, she could breathe again. She felt her shoulders soften and lower from their proximity to her ears. Her chin rested and her face turned upward. She was sure her neck was longer now that she wasn't bending over a desk for hours on end. She slept in her old bed between cool crisp line-dried sheets, the windows opened with delicate white ruffled Cape Cod curtains softly moving in the night breeze. Familiar smells of farmer's fields in the fall, earth turned to prepare for spring, sounds of Amish clip clopping down rural roads, or a stream running icy cold over the smooth rock lining the creek. Birds sang by day.

The cardinal's whistle, the blue jay's persistent call, the chickadees and sparrows and tufted titmouse all at play around Aunt Diane's bird feeders. Denny had forgotten how many varieties she recognized by their song from the hours her aunt had spent with her as a child. Aunt Diane and Aunt Rita had raised Denny at least as much as Helen had. Helen off to trainings to be a doula, or births to attend as the midwife's apprentice, workshops out of town, overnight births that ran for days. There was no inducing a mother who chose a natural birth. Birth was in the hands of a power far more revered than an OB doctor, or even the midwife. The whole idea was to facilitate birth, not rush it or try to control it or make it conform to the timetable of man. It was sacred. Intimate. Between mother and child and the forces of God and nature. Which is why Helen was away for unpredictable lengths of time, and Denny was cared for as often by her two aunts.

As she lie in bed listening to the sound of crickets and frogs calling to each other with a plucking sound like rubber bands echoing through the night she was bathed in a soothing comfort. *Restorative*. It was a term used in her yoga classes, but never did it feel so defined as on the farm. She didn't miss the city. But she did miss Melissa. Mel was intense and animated and on this unusual occasion, ready for a party. She was gushing, and very obviously tickled that Denny had come.

They caught the early show of Phantom of the Opera, then went to Joe Allen's after for some grilled shrimp and roasted salmon, eating light so they wouldn't be sleepy for the party. Mel could hardly contain her excitement being with Denny. She was sure her dearest friend was about to encounter her future husband. She had done her research on the famous Bishop Belanger and his son Maxwell and their collaborative architecture firm in Canada. She had checked out Max and lingered over his photo on their firm's web page.

"He's quite attractive," Mel said to Denny. "I told my friend from the MET that she *must* introduce us."

Oh jeez. What have I gotten myself into. Denny sighed.

Denny spotted him across the room, leaning with one arm on the fireplace mantle, a rocks glass in his hand, swirling ice cubes and talking with a shapely brunette whose dress was a couple sizes too small for her figure. She may have been able to pull it off had she worn some kind of shapewear underneath, but instead, she was squeezed in and oozing out in all the wrong places like a zip-tied monkey sock. Aside from that, her face looked soft enough and she was clearly interested in whatever the architect was saying.

He was tall and slender and dressed like an older gentleman professor. Nobody Denny's age wore corduroys. His were a chocolate shade of brown and resembled a nice pair of slacks. They were fitted like a sleeve down his long legs that went on forever, to his bare ankles and soft worn leather loafers. He wore no socks, which gave him a casual look, like maybe wearing shoes at all was an afterthought. His full head of rich brown hair was tied back at the nape of his neck, with just a few inches in a ponytail. Not a single strand of hair was out of place, but there was no slick look to his locks. It was just pulled back like Antonio Banderas, or Brad Pitt. Clean shiny, off the face revealing beautifully sculpted features. His jawline was sharp with a prominent turn under his earlobe and a muscle that flexed in his jaw when he wasn't talking. Denny thought she might like to let his hair out of that ponytail. He wore a leather vest a shade or two lighter than his corduroys. It didn't match the pants; but was more an accessory. She could almost picture him with a medieval pirate shirt beneath the vest, but what he actually wore was a simple fitted cashmere sweater the color of milk, pushed up to the elbows, revealing nice, chiseled forearms. *Intriguing*, she thought, enjoying his style. A combination of artist, surfer and sophisticate. No one she knew dressed like that.

As it turned out, no one had to introduce them. He made his way over to Denny after she and Mel had met the host and mingled a little bit. When Denny turned to get a drink, there he was. He spoke softly, a bit shy maybe. But with a confidence and posture that made him alluring.

"I took a chance you might like to start with champagne?" He held out a glass and smiled warmly. "I'm Max." She took the glass from him with a nod and as soon as their eyes met, she knew that she would indeed marry this architect.

Chapter 3

The wedding was affectionately referred to as shotgun for the rest of their lives. Their romance was a whirlwind and Denny was completely dumfounded by the unexpected spell she was under. She had never been in love at all, she decided. Anything she'd ever felt before Max was now overshadowed the way a blade of grass is overshadowed by a giant oak tree. There was no comparison. She was humbled to discover how happy she could be, and by surrendering completely to the powerful love she was feeling her days were filled with pleasure. And the pregnancy? It thrilled her. She was frequently opening her mouth and inserting a fork full of all the declarations she had made up until then: She would never marry, she didn't want children, she would never rely on a man, she would be his equal if a man was allowed along for the ride at all. She would always have a career. She would never be stuck as a homemaker. On and on she was humbled. Again and again eating her words. But neither Helen nor her Aunt Rita were surprised. Goldenrod was in love. And when that happens, all bets are off. She had not bargained for the power of Max Belanger. He turned her world upside down and uncovered desires she didn't know she had. She could hardly believe what was happening. She really *did* want eight babies and a life in rural Canada in a log cabin with her architect. It made her head swim. And whenever she felt a little nudge in her abdomen, the fluttering new life inside, she chuckled with delight at the insanity of it.

They drove the 3,600 miles from the farm in Croghan to Whitehorse Yukon, across the country through Minnesota, North Dakota, through the Great Plains, which neither thought were very great. But once on the northern trek into Canada, the pristine green lakes and jutting mountain scenery took Denny's breath away. Crossing into Saskatchewan, they stopped in Moose Jaw, then on to Edmonton and Watson Lake, finally arriving in Whitehorse, where Max had grown up. The trip took a week and a half, and the newlyweds were dancing on air barely noticing they had crossed an entire continent. Denny was only sick once, after a prenatal vitamin with a coffee chaser on an empty stomach. Max had to pull the car over in a hurry and that was the only incident of morning sickness the entire pregnancy.

For Max, the journey back to Canada, was a long time coming. He had established himself in his father's company and was already an accomplished architect when Denny began her life with him. His schedule was relentless, his ambition energizing. He worked with the Smithsonian, student centers, rehab centers, churches, cathedrals, schools, colleges, city halls, and on and on the list went. He was well accomplished, receiving honors from countless groups. Gold medal awards, crystal globe awards, WoodWorks awards, achievement awards, mason design awards, best building awards, prizes for the arts, just to name a few.

However well intended, he did not settle down to raise a family. Quite the opposite. Denny quickly discovered her architect husband could only remain on top of his game if he kept moving. And move he did. First he moved her to Whitehorse where, just as she had allegedly predicted, they bought a gorgeous eight bedroom, five bath log cabin. It was over the top, and Denny nearly dug in her heels to refuse, but his excitement won her over.

"We're getting started on eight kids, love. We're going to need the room! And I'm going to need a house big enough that I can get you away from them and we can keep having honeymoon sex," He grabbed her, pulling her close, careful not to bump her growing mid-section. "You are so sexy when you're pregnant! I could get used to this."

Denny was blissful to be expecting, and even happier to be enjoying her Max. It was a challenge to get his time, as he was always working on something, or traveling for a job. She managed to step back and not take it personally. She was proud of him and his passion. It was part of what drew her to him. His style, and quirkiness and creativity. She compared him to Hemingway, or Howard Hughes. He was her very own eccentric tortured artist who is all at once fascinating, and infuriating. Beautiful, and selfish. Artistic and depressed. He kept her on her toes with his continual mood shifts and spontaneous trips out of town. It could have been a disaster, having all those babies with an absentee dad, but her life was full. And she had found something she loved to do. Being a mother was a role she felt innately suited for. She was challenged, nurtured, and fulfilled, and thankfully, Max relished fatherhood too. Denny intended their firstborn to be named for Max. They had refused ultrasounds and had no idea their little Max would be a girl. His eyes filled up with tears after the birth and he exclaimed, "Oh my God. That was amazing! Let's do it again!"

Thus, Denny weaned her firstborn, Maxine when she was just four months old so they could get pregnant again. And just thirteen months after Maxine was born, came their second child, Helena. Before long, a decade had passed, and Max and Denny had five gorgeous kids. Maxine, Helena, Amber, Alex, and Bishop.

First Maxine, (they both liked the idea of Max for a girl, so it stuck). Helena was named for Denny's mom, and Amber for Max's mom. Alex and Bishop were named after their grandfathers, even though they too, were baby girls, and Joe was the boy that came at last.

Goldenrod's babies were toe headed blondes, and by eight or ten years of age, their hair began to darken and they looked more like their father. Summers were short in the Yukon, but the children's hair would bleach out in the sun and they looked like Denny again. Maxine and Helena were so close in age, they called themselves the twins. They were asked by strangers on the street if they were twins so many times, that they approved and adopted it as truth. Though they looked amazingly similar, they were very different in personality. Maxine quickly became the responsible older sibling, and more so as siblings were added. She was the miniature mom, a fretting hen, bossy and responsible. Helena had a short attention span, plenty of energy, and gave Maxine a run for her money. Still, they were thick as thieves and joined at the hip. When Amber arrived, she followed the twins around, thumb in her mouth and observed. She was a cheery chubby cheeked child with huge eyes like a Keane painting from the seventies, but her eyes were smiling, curious, full of wonder, and blue as the sky. She mostly watched her sisters play act. They liked to set up the camera and pretend they were hosting a talk show, or they would put on a production of the Hobbit and invite the neighborhood kids to watch. Amber often brought a book to Maxine's lap and asked her what a word was. Maxine would settle in and just read her the rest of the story, or she'd help her sound out the word and send her on her way.

When Alex came along, the entertainment had arrived. She loved the spotlight, and even as a baby, if someone giggled at her antics, she would repeat them endlessly. Laughter in the Belanger house was contagious and Alex could always be counted on to get the ball rolling. She was intrigued by all sorts of talents and deeply coveted them all. Endlessly watching music videos and falling in and out of love with movie stars, pop stars, or even a friend of the family who showed up with the least bit of musical inclination, a guitar, a harmonica, a dramatic flair, or funky new fashion. Her father, being a nearly famous architect, was fascinating to her, but not nearly as fascinating as her grandfather. Bishop Belanger was on the cover of Time magazine! All of Canada knew who he was. He was even known around the world! "Someday, I'll move to Hollywood. Just wait and see," Alex repeated with determined regularity.

Max traveled for work and often got the news of a new pregnancy months into it, as Denny refused to share that news over the phone. He was filled with excitement and anticipation. Denny's mother, Helen made arrangements to come for each birth. Max was often away or traveling home when Denny was in labor. He even missed the big event twice. This wasn't an issue for Denny. She had been raised around young single birthing women, and Helen as their midwife. Birth was a womankind event and although an occasional dad might catch the baby, it was rare. Women quietly labored alone or with other women. It was what Denny grew up with. The home her mother had created was full of expecting young mothers and Helen caring for them.

Denny's births took place in the comfort of her own bathtub, with Helen downstairs looking after the little ones, or working on a knitting project. If Denny moaned or called out, Helen hurried to her side. But Denny wanted to birth alone. And would call her mom only to help her get up out of the tub or hold the baby while they made their way into the bed.

The kids knew the routine. They were to keep themselves busy and entertained until Nana Helen said it was time. Then they all made their way to their mom's bed like a holy little procession of awe-struck faces, carefully climbing onto the bed, so as not to bounce mom or baby. This was followed by lots of kissing mom and petting their new baby sibling and stroking her head; the older girls asking Denny if she was okay and if they could bring her anything. A cookie maybe? They had been making chocolate chip cookies while she labored in the tub.

Oftentimes the entire crew would sleep in the bed, or around the bed on the floor with sleeping bags when Max was away. If he was home, the birth routine had a different feel. Helen still managed to keep the mood calm, but Max was more nervous, which would slow things down a bit. Denny's attention was not as focused, and she tried to make sure Max was okay. They took walks outside, and Max tried to be good and attentive, but he would have been more comfortable in a hospital setting, with monitors and bells and whistles and those lines to watch on the roll of paper as contractions increased in intensity. It didn't matter that the intensity a woman actually *feels* has nothing to do with those measurements. And she can feel a doozy of a contraction but the silly machine says it's nothing at all. Max was a man, and men in a waiting area somewhere smoking cigars would have suited Denny just fine.

Max eventually learned to stall his homecoming just enough to miss the birth. He was there for the first two. And after that, his arrival time got later and later for each birth. But for the kids and Denny, it meant a slumber party in the master bedroom that may even go on a couple days.

Helen did laundry and meals and dishes and spent lots of time with the kids so they didn't feel overshadowed by the newcomer. Denny and Helen had time for reconnecting after Helen put the kids to bed. She told them stories of Denny when she was a little girl. She told them of the fields of Goldenrod she was named after, and the bees and farm and her sisters, their great aunts that they'd never met. She promised the little ones they would come for a visit when the snow melted. Denny had no desire to navigate an airport with her brood, and the drive without Max didn't sound appealing either. She was a homebody at heart, and said she'd come to NY when the kids were grown.

When Max finally arrived, it was a loud and exciting whirlwind. The house was amped with delight. The kids played in the snow with their dad. He went overboard with gifts and laughter that thrilled them all. He and the kids took over the kitchen and made huge breakfasts of pancakes and sausage and gravy and biscuits and marmalade jam and sparkling grape juice and fresh pineapple and fried eggs and rye toast and omelets and buttermilk. He took multiple trips to the grocery store and piled the kids in the jeep, leaving Denny and her mom and the newborn to have a bit of quiet. When he returned, there were lunch feasts of oysters and mussels and clams and since the kids knew how to make their own crackers, there were fresh baked crackers and hot spicy sauces and spreads of liverwurst on buttered sourdough, or chili and skillet corn bread. The whirlwind of Max lasted four of five days, until the wind in his sails began to cease and he slept through breakfast and drank coffee for lunch and seemed less interested in the kids. That's about the time he announced he had a flight to catch and he tussled the hair on their little heads and told them not to be sad, he'd be home again soon. But they all knew it could be weeks before they saw him again.

Chapter 4

Spring had sprung and Denny drove Maxine, Helena, and Amber to school and took Alex and Bishop to the playground out back. It would be an hour or two before the school kids would be using it, so they had the playground to themselves. When she was settled in on the bench she tied Bishop's shoes and Alex propped Bishop into the swing and gave her a gentle push, before jumping on her belly on another swing and chatting away to Bishop. Denny was supremely proud of her little brood and the way the cared for each other. Alex was only five, but she watched over Bishop as if she were the one who gave her life and brought her into the world. She knew FAR more than the poor little thing, and she took up the role of big sister from the day she was born. she was very aware of Bishop, making certain she's never left behind in the shuffle.

Helen struck up a conversation with another mom, Samantha, who had arrived with her boy. They were making small talk about the kids on the monkey bars, Denny pointing out her daughter Alex, and Sam motioning over to her son nearly the same age, Michael. "I've just taken him out of school and we'll be homeschooling in the fall," Sam told Denny. "I can't take the schedule and all the rushing around. And half the time in school, they're just watching movies, or doing field trips or busy work."

"Alex would have been in school this year, but we just missed the cut off date. I'm relieved not to have one more in school!" Denny had her hands full running kids to sporting events and an endless amount of after school activities. She didn't like the pace of her life-. Her idea of having a big family was working together on a farm, or a family business, or exploring the world together on adventures of their own making. The jerky, fragmented days of public school were wearing her down, and almost immediately, when she met Samantha, she jumped on the idea of bringing them all home and setting up their own lives. Not that she wanted to keep them from other kids, or from school, or learning, or even endless activities. But she wanted to be the one in charge, not at the mercy of a factory system with schedules and bells that relentlessly interrupt any creative ember before it could ever ignite. School was too rigid for her family.

Max had been an easy sell. When he was home, he would rant at the nonsense his poor six-year-old was working on. Denny hushed him. "Not in front of them," She signaled with a frown and a look, "They'll think you're not proud of them." But he wasn't like most fathers. He could care less about the grades they brought home. He wanted to see what *talents* they were developing, or what *passions* they had acquired. If anything, he observed that school was quenching any spirit they had. But he left the bulk of the parenting to Denny, since he had no intention of rearranging his life to be more involved at home, nor did he give much thought to any alternatives. He lit up however, when Denny told him in no uncertain terms that she would be homeschooling their children beginning in the fall. Far from cautioning or discouraging her, Max grabbed her around the hips, lifted her up and twirled her around the kitchen until she was yelling at him, too dizzy for anymore. She was relieved and a little surprised by his reaction. *That was too easy!* She thought.

"Our children are far too good for regular schooling," Max laughed and spoke with a snooty faux British accent, grabbing the mop handle to use as his cane. He tossed a plastic mixing bowl on his head for a bowler hat and shouted, "Hey! Teacher! Leave those kids alone!"

"I've been reading about the Montessori Method, my *daaawling* clever husband," Denny and Max were performing now, as all the kids had jostled into the kitchen since they heard their mother screeching to be put down.

"Monte who?" Max threw his head back, nose in the air and did his best snob impression.

"Why, dawling. Have you not heard? Maria Montessori is the mother of all child-led education!" She spoke down to him as if only a fool would not know this.

"Posh!" Max exclaimed, "And·who, pray tell is the father of…" But Denny broke in.

"Why John Holt of course! Have you been living under a rock, dear?"

"Who's John Holt," Alex was tugging on Denny's pantleg. Max picked up Alex and set her squarely on the island countertop covered with blue Mexican tiles. He spun her around to face her mother and wrapped his arms around her. With his chin resting on her little shoulder he turned his attention to Denny. With a feigned seriousness and a furrowed brow he said,

"Yes, love. Please tell us. Who is John Holt?" Alex looked at her father and then frowned intently as well, awaiting her mother's reply.

"He was a schoolteacher in the 60's that became disillusioned and decided the school system could not possibly be reformed. He then became an advocate for home schooling, and ultimately unschooling."

Alex was frowning still. "I like school. What's wrong with school?" But the older kids were cheering and asking if they could sleep in every morning and play video games all day and ditch the textbooks. In no time the kitchen was a buzz with all kids talking at once and asking a million questions. Aside from Alex and little Bishop who wasn't old enough to know what the fuss was all about, the idea was a hit.

All spring and throughout the summer, Denny researched educational philosophies. She read books like How Children Learn, Teach Your Own by Holt and Farenga, Home Grown Kids, Home Spun Schools, Better Late than Early by Raymond and Dorothy Moore. Then there were the Gatto books: Dumbing Us Down, and The Underground History of American Education. Gatto taught in New York city schools for over thirty years, won the New York State Teacher of the Year award and then promptly spoke out against the entire system of public education for the rest of his life. Denny was fully engrossed and fascinated by all of these renegade philosophers. One of the most fascinating facts from Gatto's Underground History of American Education book was the image he painted of some American elitists traveling to Prussia in the late 1700's and deciding that their system of compulsory education would work wonderfully in America, especially with our industrial revolution underway. Massachusetts was the first to pass compulsory education laws and all families would send their kids off to school or else! Or else what? Or else they would be (and were) marched to school at bayonet point.

Gatto's writing held that the worst thing for children is to be removed from their families and entrusted to state-run institutions for education and training. Denny struggled to comb through all the twists and turns and philosophies in Gatto's history lesson. It was wordy and convoluted and she would sit up late nights when everyone was asleep and try to decipher what this man was going on about. Still there was an underlying theme, a strand of truth that emerged again and again like a shiny gold thread weaving its way toward the end of the book until finally the light of dawn washed over a sleepy Denny. And suddenly she was filled with an excitement that would propel her for years to come.

A thought no less intense than the scene where the Grinch's heart grows three sizes and a halo appears above his head and his eyes fill with tears. She had a legitimate purpose. And it was all bound in the keeping and teaching and loving and training of those babies she'd brought into the world. What could matter more?

Goldenrod remembered her own childhood. She rode the school bus in the morning without question and dutifully did as she was told. But when the bus pulled up to take her little ones off to school, she found no joy or relief or even pride in it. She felt loss. She didn't want the kids out of her hair in order to do some other thing. They weren't in the way, nor were they keeping her from anything. *They* were what she wanted to do.

Her first glimpse into the world of homeschooling came when her new friend Sam invited her along to the home of another woman, Wendy. They were getting together to share ideas about curriculum, teaching methods, problems, legalities, and other nuts and bolts of home schooling.

Denny stood at the kitchen island absorbing all the smells and sounds of Wendy's home. To her left, hanging in the front window was a birdcage full of little zebra finches chattering away with quiet songs and peeps that sound like the tiniest horns playing. There were two friendly mutt dogs sniffing around at her pantlegs with wagging tails. A kid about nine or ten came bounding down the stairs with a worksheet in his hand and thrust it at Wendy saying, "She got em all right but two," and then he ran off and back up the stairs skipping every other step as he went.

Wendy had retrieved the paper and was looking for a place to set it down, since the counters were covered with flour. There were two pajama clad girls at work in the kitchen rolling out dough into thin sheets and pricking them with a fork.

"You'll have to excuse the mess," she said apologetically, "they wanted to make crackers."

People make crackers? Denny thought, trying to take it all in. She had never thought of Saltines from anywhere but the grocery store. *Who makes crackers?* These people had nowhere to go, nowhere they had to be. They *lived* here. There was no sense of rushing around to get out the door. There was no pressure to stay on schedule. What day is it anyway? Isn't it Tuesday? It's like a Saturday here, or a summer vacation.

Denny was immediately reminded of her mother's kitchen; the warm bowls of rising bread everywhere, the girls on the farm learning to milk goats and make soap, doing chores or peeling apples with her Aunt Diane, learning to make a pie crust, and always having something warm on the stove. Denny looked around at this woman's home, and the carefree way her kids were living, and she knew immediately what she would do for the next 20 years.

Denny started ordering curriculum, workbooks, and even wall décor; an alphabet in cursive for around the top of the kitchen walls, some charts and posters and maps began to appear on the log walls of the home. The youngest kids were excited, the older kids relieved, but Alex was vacillating back and forth between excitement and a sense of loss. She really liked the social aspect of school. She loved her teacher dearly, and her friends even more. There was plenty of drama for a girl in second grade. Who was whose best friend changed each day, leaving a wake of heartbreak. Alex had come home with new dramas every day about this friend or that friend who liked the boy she liked or the trouble she was in for passing a note during a social studies lesson. Denny knew Alex thrived on the drama, but didn't think it would be detrimental to her development to replace it all with Home Ec.

Chapter 5

Max clenched his jaw and groaned as he waited for his flight. His head was throbbing and his mouth felt like it was stuck shut from dryness. His eyes were heavy as if some clawed thing was sitting on his scalp pushing all the flesh from his forehead to his eyelids. He was angry and miserable and didn't know why. Which was only adding to the misery. He had gone back and forth, trying to be home longer this time. He could see the disappointment in Denny and the kids. But it seemed the damn moods were catching up to him. Hot on his trail with relentless pursuit, and running was all he knew to do.

Max was down. And when he was down, it was time to go. This wasn't a new routine. His misery would drive him to a hotel room somewhere in the lower forty-eight, where he put himself to bed. Sometimes for a couple days. Sometimes for a week.

"Now boarding flight 559 Air North to Vancouver," the echo of a loudspeaker interrupted his funk and jaw clenching. Max picked up his bag and watched the diamond shapes on the carpet as he made his way to the ticket agent at the gate. He thrust his ticket toward her and said nothing when she greeted him and wished him a good flight. He never looked up. His head hurt. His body felt like it was under a thousand extra pounds. The only relief in sight was the thought that in less than twenty-four hours he'd be laying in a bed in the dark. Max hadn't lied when he told his family he had to get back to work. He had a small project in Chicago he was working on. Thankfully, his dad had the lead on the project, and Max was just support. And of course his dad did not need support. In fact, he and his dad were butting heads at every turn, Max wanting to bring his own creative concepts to the table, and his dad snowplowing ahead without hearing him. This wasn't unusual. And this is why they rarely worked together anymore. Their collaborations usually did not end well, and Max had hesitated to get involved in this project, but he needed the money, and he had other reasons to be in Chicago.

The flight attendant appeared offering some prepackaged cookies and soda and alcohol options. Max traveled so often that he had this part down to a science. Get all the nips and shooters they'll allow and pocket a few for the cab ride to the hotel. He ordered a coke and five nips of Jack Daniels. He put two in his drink, and three in his pocket. Then he drank it down quick and put his head back to hopefully get some sleep until he could get to where he would sleep some more. As he closed his eyes and the plane hummed like a giant grasshopper over the clouds, he thought about his Goldenrod and how beautiful she was. He sighed with disappointment. *Stuck with me,* he thought. *She deserves more.* He was dead weight. She was lovely, innocent and tired. *Why doesn't she just unhinge herself from this farce of a human being. Why does she stay with me.*

And then he recalled all those adorable baby faces that were his very own offspring. The tow-headed bundles of squishy goodness. And again, he shook his head. *Uh. And me for a father. Jesus. The poor things.*

When Max got to his hotel room in Chicago, his mood hadn't improved. He was so sick of himself, sick of his thoughts, sick of his self-loathing, self-pitying self that he wanted to die. He went to bed and prayed for death to come.

Denny didn't complain that Max had left her again. He was a very big presence when he was home. Everything revolved around him. It was impossible to just go on with a quiet routine. Once Max arrived, all normalcy was out the window. He was loud. He was animated. He was magnetic. The kids would orbit him with an innate attraction no less resistible than gravity and motion. She too, was under his spell and happy he was home, for however long it would last. But she knew it wouldn't last. The jobs he did, the crazy hours he kept, the projects that were high pressure and larger than life, the constant travel, the hero he played when he was home, it was all his way of surviving. Keep moving. Fly high. But what goes up, must come down eventually. And come down he would. Then he would leave. She still pictured him standing against that fireplace at a party in New York, his artsy look and his charming presence. The hottest architect in Canada. She knew even then that he was not to be molded or shaped into her life. But she had an uncanny desire to be part of his. And she was delighted to be making babies with him.

Chapter 6

Max slept solid over the next few days. The do-not- disturb sign dangled from the handle of his door and the drapes were drawn over closed blinds. A loud steady hum from the fan in the wall unit kept him unaware of any noise outside the room. He got up by the dim light of the bedside clock and used the bathroom half asleep. Eventually he got restless and fished around for his phone. Four voicemails from his dad. One from Clarissa. *Better get some coffee and a shower before I listen to those.* He groaned, turned on a bedside lamp and looked at the digital clock on the nightstand. 2:22. *Sounds ominous. AM or PM,* he wondered. He got up and opened the drapes and blinds to discover a rainy, slushy, wet snow kind of day. He sighed and thought about getting back to his dark hole under the covers. But he was done with sleep. And his cranium was splitting from caffeine withdrawal.

Room service was at the door as he was shaving. The shower felt good, but the coffee couldn't come quick enough. He ordered an entire pot with some breakfast croissants, jelly, scrambled eggs and a double order of sausage patties. On second thought, make that a double order of everything.

Max spread out his portfolio and looked over the plans and dates he had arranged with his father. He had only been asleep since Thursday.

Slept through the weekend and part of Monday. Now he had to rejoin the living. His father had arranged an unveiling of their most recent project, the Aldana Health Center in downtown Chicago. A typical black tie evening soiree with the who's who of the city including dinner, cocktails and yawns. This will be followed the next day by a ribbon cutting ceremony and open house for the press and general public. Max was dreading both. But he was relieved to be finished with the joint work with his father.

With half a sausage patty in his mouth, he checked his messages with dread. From his father, "Max. It would be nice if you would check in with me and let me know you've made it to Chicago."

"Uh, Max. Your phone die or something? We are ON for Thursday's opening. We need to get together and go over the last-minute details, press talk, you know the drill. Call me."

"Max. What the hell. It's Monday and I still haven't heard from you. You better have your shit together for Thursday,"

And then,

"Hi Max. It's Clarissa. I expected to hear from you by now. I know you have an unveiling this week, and we need to talk. Please call me,"

Max finished his breakfast in silence thinking about Clarissa. He hadn't spoken with her in years, and out of the blue, she's wanting to connect. Their affair was a brief one. She was working for the mayor at the time, and the building project couldn't be settled on, despite the wining and dining the city was doing to enlist his expertise. Max and his father were overloaded with a couple other projects and simply couldn't squeeze in a health center. Especially when the size and scope of the project was so small. It would take time away from the big money to be made on a multimillion-dollar project. But once things quieted and other projects were wrapped up, they found time to return to Chicago and do this one last project together. And Max made it clear that this would be their last one. Max had been living in the shadow of his father for a while now, and he was ready to break out on his own.

Clarissa was in those initial meetings years ago, and the fire between them was irresistible. Max played his usual charming artist routine, and she was coming on strong. He wasn't proud of his infidelities, but he managed to live with himself with some lame justifications. He was on the road. He was lonely. He was a man. He was crazy about Denny and had no interest in trading her in. She was the love of his life. But Max wasn't very skilled in denying himself. When Clarissa invited him to her room, he went.

Now he was sitting at the River Roast watching the door. He had called his Dad and reassured him that all was well and yes, he was in Chicago, and yes, he's ready for Thursday night. He called Denny a second time. He never missed a message letting her know he'd arrived. Or that he was heading back. But they usually didn't talk much when he was away. She was engrossed with the kids, and he was busy with work…mostly. She suspected he crashed a bit when they were apart, but she didn't know the extent of the funk he sunk to. He didn't share it. He didn't want to know about it or think about it himself, so he certainly wasn't going to fill her in.

A woman came in the door and quickly made eye contact with Max, but he didn't recognize her. However, she headed straight toward him and started to sit down. Max jumped up realizing this was a very different Clarissa. He pulled the chair our for her and helped her take her coat off. Then he found a coatrack and hung it and he returned to her. Her eyes never left him. He sat across from her, disturbed and troubled. He tried not to let it show on his face. "Clarissa," he spoke softly.

"I'm sorry if I scared you."

"No, don't be ridiculous. It's just that…"

"Pancreatic cancer. I'm dying Max."

That much was obvious. He was shocked at the ashy gray color of her face, even her lips. And the bones around her eyes and cheeks looked like they were fighting to get out of her skin. She had hair, but as he looked more closely, he could see that it was a wig. She reached up self-consciously to scratch or adjust it. It was too big for her tiny skull.

The waitress came to his rescue and Max ordered a beer. Clarissa drank water and Max asked awkwardly if she was able to eat anything? When she chuckled a little bit, something in the way her face moved reminded Max of an animated skeleton from a cereal commercial. He was intently focusing on keeping his face expressionless. It was hard work.

"I'll have the market soup and the mushroom toast," she told the waitress. Her voice was raspy and slight, like her body. But the waitress stood staring at her. The place was noisy. Max decided maybe she didn't hear. Either that or she was stupefied by the talking skeleton sitting at the table. So he repeated,

"The MARKET SOUP, and MUSHROOM TOAST" Then he said, "I'LL HAVE THE SAME." She snapped out of her daze and hurried off without grabbing the menus.

Max didn't know what to say. "I'm so sorry Clarissa."

"Don't be. You didn't do anything,"

He sat wondering why she had called him. Why would she want to see him if she's dying. It was hard not to stare. What was once long jet-black hair, thick and shiny like a mane on a Frisian show horse, was now a short wig, too big for her head. And her thick umber skin that fit tight like a glove, shiny and dark and rich, was now ashen with bruises around her wrists, disappearing up the sleeve where he was sure there were more. Her body had been full and thick and beautiful, like that of an exotic island belly dancer with long eyelashes and a bracelet high on her arm, over her bicep. Yet here she sat like wrinkled wrapping paper left over from a gift long gone. It was filling him with deep sorrow. Not that she had been a gorgeous creature. Not the vanity of her beauty or her sexuality and appeal. But the fact that the very life she was so full of had completely vanished without a trace, leaving in its wake this animated skeleton person. Even her eyes were hollow. He tried to make conversation to break the silence. "How long have you been sick?"

"About a year and a half," she was trembling as she took small sips from her water glass. Max thought of the water coming out from between her ribs like a sprinkler. He bit his lip and chided himself for his stupid thoughts. He was beginning to wish he hadn't ordered any food because he wanted to get out of there. He began to watch the door and think of ways he could slip out. Her back was to the door. He could excuse himself to use the restroom and then just leave. She wouldn't see.

The waitress appeared with their food and asked Max if he'd like another beer.

"No thanks, I'm good." As she walked away he groaned thinking of the check. He could slip out of this awful lunch, but he wasn't cruel enough to leave her with the check. She sat quietly sipping her soup in slow motion. And suddenly Max couldn't stand being there for another second. He excused himself to head for the bathroom, and nearly knocked over his waitress as he rushed by. He took her arm to steady her and whispered, "Hey, listen. Tell the lady at the table I had an emergency, will ya? And this should cover our lunch," he handed her a wad of cash and as he hurried out of the River Roast, he looked over his shoulder to see the waitress heading over to Clarissa.

Chapter 7

Clarissa had nearly lost her mind. Dying gave her permission to think and live and behave in ways she had never dreamed of before. Nothing mattered anymore. No opinions or estimations from others, no judgements, no guilt, no holding back. She could be as honest or as deceptive as she wanted to be. God owed her that. If he was going to take away her life, he at least couldn't judge her for how she spent what was left of it. She looked herself over in the mirror and shuddered to think how cruel cancer had been to her body. But rather than cry or surrender to defeat, she smashed the mirror to bits and found her most glamorous fitted sequin gown, the blue one she wore the night she seduced Max.

It didn't fit snug anymore. In fact, it was hanging too long and too low. The long V in the back plunged nearly to her skinny tailbone. The sexy halter neckline draped over her sharp protruding clavicle bones and puckered where her breasts used to be. She threw a cashmere shawl of the same deep rich blue over her shoulders and convinced herself she was still the captivating enchantress she had always been.

Clarissa was born in Jamaica. Her mum was a very light-skinned Jamaican, her dad's dad was English and her dad's mum was Portuguese. The rest of the family was Jamaican. She came to the United States as an adolescent passing herself off as an adult. She had street smarts from years of navigating her own survival, for although she had parents, they were mostly unavailable to her. She was left too often with an overly helpful uncle who volunteered to keep her. As early as her ninth birthday he had terrorized her into posing nude and forced her to make videos holding weapons to her throat threatening to carve her up like a turkey if she were to ever tell what they were up to in their private sessions. He had cut the family dog in front of her for good measure.

Clarissa became tough as nails. She turned all of her fear and anger and misfortune into a steel will to not only survive, but to become the sexiest and most powerful woman in the world. She would flip the tables and turn her beauty into a skill set that would land her in places so high, she could never fall again. And her uncle? One day she would return to take care of him the way he took care of the dog.

After her daughter was born, she softened a bit, never forgetting where she came from, but growing a kinder heart as time went on. Six years earlier, Max was just another easy target for her love games. She always went for the most powerful man in the room. But on this occasion, she chose the younger architect over his father. They were both good looking men. But Max was striking. And she was like a black widow spider licking her lips at the sight of him. The men she had seduced over the years were men of great means who she could blackmail after their brief affair. She had learned all the tricks, hiding cameras and getting the best angles and sound recordings while she was being educated by her uncle. He made a fortune on her selling kiddy porn online and all the while, she was taking notes, determined to make it count. Every single wretched episode, every moment, every ounce of pain and shame and disgust, she would turn into a skill that would benefit and empower her. She swore to herself that she would get back to Jamaica and kill him one day. It made her nauseous to think he got away with all he had done to her.

Clarissa never blackmailed Max after their little fling. Maybe it was all those kids he had, or maybe it was his sensitivity during their time together. He hadn't rushed to get her clothes off when they arrived in her room. He hadn't acted like a dog in heat, or a pervert or a stupid clumsy boy. He sat quietly and stared at her curiously. She had teasingly undressed for him the way she had for dozens of men. But unlike the others, he just looked at her with a warmth and patience that confused her. She felt vulnerable and exposed, instead of powerful and confident. For a moment, when their eyes met, she nearly blushed. With a nervous cover of playfulness, she jumped under the sheets and watched Max. Locking eyes with hers, he undressed and slipped between the covers with her, pulling her close. He kissed her softly with his eyes open, like he didn't want to miss anything. With his head on the pillow he watched her face. For a minute, she thought maybe he was going to fall asleep. Everything was moving too slow. She felt off her game. *Snap out of it! What is this?* She wanted to curl up and cuddle in this man's warmth rather than have any sex at all. *But NO, No way. This is bullshit. I didn't bring him up here to snuggle! No this guy's my ticket to retirement.*

Then she was on top of him and she morphed into the skillful, licentious lover she had become over years of practice. She transported Max to a place of uninhibited ecstasy until something was just a little too wonderful. And a creepy feeling quietly intruded on his pleasure hinting that whatever this was, it was too good to be true and he shouldn't trust her.

Jada was born thirty-eight weeks later. The pregnancy was a turning point for Clarissa. She had accumulated plenty of money, much of it coming in regular monthly payments for the lifetime of the "doners", and though this pregnancy caught her off guard, she felt it was a sign. An opportunity to get on a straight path. Clarissa had a soft spot for Max. The night she brought him home, he had broken the barrier of disdain she held for all men since she was just a little girl. Somehow he tore a little hole in it. And some warm feelings that were new and foreign to her came through. It wasn't an explosion, or even a gust. But it was an opening. And it wobbled her foundation like the tremor of a small earthquake.

When she discovered she was pregnant, Clarissa deleted all the footage she had of their escapade in the hotel room. Max had no way of knowing Jada even existed, and she had no intention of telling him. She would hold all the cards and all the responsibility of this new life.

Chapter 8

Max stood looking out at the city lights and thinking of his Denny. He felt like he was returning from the dark place and wished he were home. She was his compass. His true north. She understood him and accepted him even though they never discussed it. *Warts and all,* he thought. *She loves me warts and all.*

The cocktail reception had just begun and Max was thinking he couldn't bear to stay all evening. He had had the awkward words with his father and put on the phony charm for the guests. He was feeding off all the buzz and admiration, and actually did feel a little better than when he'd first arrived in Chicago. Aside from that weird lunch with Clarissa, things were looking up. The venue was an elaborate event space with windows overlooking the city. The glass staircase leading to the cocktail lounge was lit from beneath creating a modern romantic effect.

When Clarissa arrived in the lobby the tall glass staircase was the first thing she noticed. She had never been to this venue before and was short of breath just from walking from the car that valet had moved. When the coat check helped her with her long formal fur, he held his breath to prevent the gasp. He was stunned by the bones of her shoulder blades protruding from her back, the elbows and shoulders looked to be painfully pushing through the skin. She gave him a slow nod and walked toward the glass stairs. One by one, she clicked her heels on the steps, gripping the

clear resin banister. She paused looking up and willed herself to continue
as if it were a great mountain climb she had prepared her entire life for. At
last, she reached the top and scanned the room looking for Max. There
near the windows to her right she discovered him. He was easy to find in a
crowd. Six or eight people were gathered around him and laughing. He
was exactly this entertaining the night she met him, six years before. The
scene was the same, and she had casually walked up and blended in to
listen. But she knocked him off his game with her beauty, and he began to
stumble and stutter and lose track of his story telling. She decided she
would just approach him again in the same way she had when they met.
But just as she stretched her foot out to take the first step toward Max, the
whole world made a humming sound and her peripheral vision began to
darken, closing in more and more as her head felt lighter and her eyes
rolled back into her head and she slumped to the floor like a tiny pile of
pick-up sticks.

The whole room gasped and one woman was over her immediately
checking her pulse and yelling, "Someone call for an ambulance! Now!"

Max looked over to see what the disturbance was, but he only saw a
cluster of people and couldn't see what was happening. The room was
hushed, and people stayed where they were, talking quietly until the
paramedics arrived. When finally, the cluster dispersed to make room for
the stretcher, Max saw the skeletal waif of a person they were moving.
And he knew at once it was Clarissa, and she had come for him. He
excused himself from the other guests and quietly followed a distance
behind the paramedics. When they had loaded her into the ambulance, and
were about to shut the door, he asked, "Can I ride along to the hospital?"

"Are you family?"

"No. I'm not. She came to see me today. I'm a friend."

"Sorry man. We're taking her to Northwest if you want to follow us
there." Max felt the slam of the door go through him. A few taxi cabs were

parked outside the venue. "Follow the ambulance to Northwest," Max said as he jumped in the back. He sighed deeply and wondered what Clarissa had been doing in a formal gown at tonight's event. He had left her at lunch in a cowardly move like no other. But she was so hard to look at. And he never did learn why she wanted to meet him. Now he felt guilty and a little responsible. He sat in the waiting room of the ER wondering if anyone else would come for her. He didn't know enough about her to know who to call, or if there even was anyone to call. He remembered she was from Jamaica. And her uncle was a creep. But those were the only details he could think of. After several hours of no news, he approached the desk and asked if he could see Clarissa or the doctor who was taking care of her. He was told to have a seat and someone would be right out. When a tall thin intern came from the back, he spoke briefly with the nurse behind the desk, who pointed to Max.

Max rose to greet him and they shook hands. "Are you the husband?"

"No, sir. I'm a friend."

"Well, what can you tell me about the patient?"

"I just met with her today, and she told me she had pancreatic cancer. Before that, I haven't seen her for years."

"Do you know if she has any family in the area?"

"Not really, Doc. I'm sorry. I may not be of much help. Is she going to be okay?"

"Well, no. I don't think she has much time left at all. But she is in and out of consciousness, and maybe you could talk to her and see if there is someone we can call."

And with that, the doctor led Max into the curtained area where Clarissa lie. Her evening gown had been replaced with a hospital gown, and she was wearing oxygen and had an IV. Max nodded at the doc who left the room. He approached the bed, leaned over and put a hand on Clarissa's gently.

"Can you hear me Clarissa?" Max was mustering up all his nerve because he didn't want to be there, nor did he think he belonged there. She opened her eyes and pulled her oxygen mask down below her chin.

"Please call my sister, Max. Her number is in my phone. Emergency contacts. It's not locked." Then she closed her eyes again, like that little sentence took a lot of work, and she pulled the oxygen back up over her mouth.

Max called the number and the woman on the other end sounded frantic. She hung up quickly once Max told her where Clarissa was. He sat down and waited. He looked at his own phone and thought about calling Denny. But he didn't know what to say. And for a moment he was grateful they didn't talk much when he was away. The calls felt awkward, and it just seemed easier to both of them to live their separate lives. Being on the phone but not together just made the distance seem greater. Denny pretended Max was out to sea, or on a secret mission, or in some far away land where there were no phones. They rarely called each other. Sometimes for weeks. But they would send little love texts now and then. And if one of them wanted to, they could call.

As Max scrolled through his old messages from Denny, the clock on the wall ticked loudly. He wondered if these were the last moments for Clarissa. He hoped her sister would arrive soon, as he didn't want to be the one with her when she died. Poor thing. Stuck in a hospital bed with nobody but him. He felt small and lame again. A swish of the curtain startled him and the doc was back with a worried looking gray haired woman holding the hand of a little girl who looked to be about six. The girl tore away from the woman shouting, "Muma!" and climbed up on the bed hugging her mother and touching her face with her hand. Clarissa opened her eyes and stroked her girl's head and kissed her gently, all the while, looking at Max.

"This is what I was wanting to tell you, Max," She managed to whisper. "Say hello to Jada," and then with her lips she mouthed *your daughter*.

45

Chapter 9

Denny had given up on the idea of ever becoming a family of church regulars on Sunday mornings. But she tried. The fire of faith inside made her want to connect with others who felt the same. Which is why she didn't fit in on Sunday mornings with the protestants. Very nice folks, but no deeper questioning, no fire, Spirit, or any of the stuff she was so enthralled by. These people were perfectly satisfied. Satisfied to show up once a week and see their friends and family. Hear a message, maybe have a potluck. Satisfied to sing from the hymnals, always at the same pace. The jubilant songs too slow, the worship songs too fast, so that none of them had the impact they were written to inspire. How could Joy to the World sound any more flat? Then the reading; a nervous soul would rise and do a scripture reading in a way that would make his high school speech teacher roll over in her grave. Had he forgotten everything? Use those nerves to enhance your speaking! Stand up straight! Speak with authority. It was the same in the Presbyterians, the Episcopalians, the Methodists, the Lutherans. Denny saw them all as very nice people. But they were not asking how to know God better. How do we get him to show up? How do we interact with the One who heals the deaf, mute, blind, lepers, paralyzed and epileptics…who causes earthquakes, falling stars, bloody moons, resurrections, angelic appearances and multiplies fish and bread. The one in the desert appearing as a pillar of fire, or a cloud to follow. Denny half wished she could just fit in. Instead, she'd been zapped by the Jesus-Red Letter Bible-Holy Ghost Power-New Birth-Pentecost fire, and she was changed. Forever. Not of her own doing. She never would have dreamed she'd become a Bible-thumper. No way. She couldn't stand those *"Have you declared Jesus Christ as your personal Lord and Savior?"* people. She cringed to think what Melissa would say of her newfound faith. She would have chosen to become something way cooler. Like a Buddhist monk, or a spiritual philosopher, or an Eastern guru of some kind. Jesus was the least fashionable to follow. She was born in the wrong time. If she could have been around for the 70's Jesus movement, when He made the cover of Time magazine and all the hippies were converting from LSD to Christ, well, that may have been cool. But now? Christianity had become a very distasteful batch of buzz words like Fundamentalists, or Evangelicals, or right wing. Terms that don't really refer to Jesus at all. Denny fell in love with the funeral-rocking, sandal-wearing, long haired Arab Jesus, by no shift of her own. It happened *TO* her. Over a kitchen table with her friend Wendy.

The stories of the gospels and the book of Acts were completely adventurous with no resemblance whatsoever to a Sunday morning in church. The normalcy choked her. The lack of expectation for anything supernatural grieved her. So she bounced around, attended lots of revival meetings, home meetings, prayer meetings, a couple of tent meetings, and on this particular occasion, from an ad she read in the paper, an invitation to a new church forming only fifteen or so miles away.

She rounded up her little Bible-thumper. Of her five kids, she only had one Bible buddy, Alex, who was ten. And she was either very concerned with pleasing her mom, or she actually had some fire and curiosity of her own. Denny would catch her sneaking cassette tapes of her favorite preacher who doubled as a comedian. Alex stayed up all night with her mom for time of fasting and prayer. Denny had read somewhere that losing sleep and staying hungry could help you experience God. Since Max was out of town, Denny and the kids prepared to stay up all night and listen to worship music and pray. The kids were excited about not going to bed. They brought their sleeping bags and pillows and claimed their spots in the living room. Maxine and Helena took one sofa, Amber, Bishop took the second sofa, and Alex looked at them curiously because she had no intention of sleeping. Their bedtime was fairly routine, but this night, their mom actually *wanted* them up all night. Alex helped her mom choose songs and scriptures to begin the night with. The rest of the kids got quiet and comfortable except for a rumpus over space on the couch. Amber and Bishop were wrestling for more room and Maxine finally shoved them off the couch and threw their bedding to the floor where they fell fast asleep.

But Alex was as determined as her mom. Not exactly sure what they hoped to accomplish, but the goal was to stay awake, so they kept right on singing, praying, and reading aloud. They kept each other up, changing worship songs to more upbeat ones, when one of them got sleepy or nodded off.

Finally, the dawn began to break and Denny whispered for Alex to follow her to the big sliding glass doors off the kitchen and watch the sun come over the horizon, bathing them with relief. It felt important. Denny thought they had done something pretty great, she and Alex. Not sure what. But cooking sausage and stacks of pancakes was their reward, and the rest of the gang awoke to a hot breakfast.

Alex came along with her mom to the new church. They didn't know what to expect, but it wasn't a crowd. There were six, or maybe less people there. The pastor, his assistant, his wife, and a couple other locals who must have seen the ad.

The church was a stately old historical building that had been there forever. But like a lot of churches in the nineties, it had closed up and was listed for sale. The brick structure was beautiful, a looming tower off one side gave it a castle effect. Inside the walls were lined with original stained-glass windows, cathedral domed ceilings, rounded archways, marble flooring and columns. There were repairs being made, some scaffolding the pastor apologized for. But then he was up front, ready to go.

Pastor Jacob was a round guy with a nicely trimmed white beard and mustache. He would have made a good Santa. He had the warmth, but he wasn't especially jovial. He was more serious and studious, wearing clergy robes with kippah and tallit, which Denny and Alex would later learn was a prayer shawl. Here was a guy with something to say. As it turned out, Denny had a great deal to learn about the Jewish roots of her Jesus. And this guy was just the man to open the doors.

Ever since her Holy Ghost "baptism", she had questioned nearly everything about her life. The homeschooling guru Wendy, was also a believer who had gently shared with Denny, inviting and challenging her to study the Bible. One of their tableside discussions ended with an "encounter" which Denny found difficult to explain. But later decided it was the Holy Spirit Baptism. Her new faith changed everything. What to do about holidays? What to do about music and movies and entertainment? How do we raise our children? What is most important? How was Jesus raised? What were His customs and routines? And of course, in a way, she thought they should just *be* Jewish! Not so much for the laws, and rules and weird stipulations against blending fabrics (from Leviticus) or the bizarre hairstyles that resemble the Amish (scenes from the wailing wall), but the *culture* of Son of God was one of great devotion and tradition, and customs.

Denny had been raised with a some of these, as a Catholic. After all, they knew about Passover. They celebrated Holy Thursday before Good Friday. She was sure if she dug in, she would find even more Jewish roots.

After the man with the unusual robe in the front of the church apologized for the repairs underway, he introduced his sidekick, who was dressed in a regular guy's suit. Navy, baggy legs, a little too long in the sleeves. White shirt. Outdated tie. He looked to be about forty and average in every way. His hair was dark and boxy, trimmed and styled in a boyish way as if his grandmother combed it for him before church every Sunday morning of his entire life, and now it was just habit. But this wasn't Sunday morning. It was Friday night; another reason Denny was keen to check it out. What kind of Christians have church on a Friday night?

When the gray-haired man began his discourse, his intelligence was immediately evident. He was articulate, charismatic, and uncommonly zealous for Christ. He was animated when he described Him on his white horse wearing a robe dipped in blood with a name written on his thigh *King of Kings and Lord of Lords*. Denny had mused that the depiction in Revelation meant that Jesus had a tattoo. But the preacher explained how the tallit would have those words written on them, and the fringe of this garment is what would be dipped in blood. This was profound and new to Denny. She wanted a lot more of this insight. He knew what he was talking about. And he was on fire.

Alex and Denny were both captivated by his preaching. And when he was finished, the small group was given a tour of the church. He expounded on his love for old, abandoned churches and his vision for the area. It was all very "happening". Much more so than the sleepy prayer meeting in the living room where they had struggled to stay awake but weren't sure why.

After the tour, the small group gathered at the back of the sanctuary pouring soda into foam cups and making little plates of Club crackers and cookies. Denny made a plate for Alex and handed her a cup of Pepsi, and then got one for herself. They stood together snacking on the fudge striped cookies, when a couple of the local guys began to argue about doctrine.

One was convinced that if you never went to church you were hell-bound. The other guy argued it was just as valid to commune with God over your fishing rod on Sunday mornings. Alex was wide eyed and her head went from side to side like she was watching a ping pong match as she listened intently to their debate. But when it heated up to lively yelling, Denny shuffled Alex out of there in a hurry. In the Jeep, she cautioned her to try to focus on the good stuff and not be bothered with that mess. Alex had pocketed some cookies for her siblings. She helped herself to one on the quiet ride home.

Chapter 10

Max's knees were trembling as he stepped backwards slowly, his eyes fixed on this little girl with her gaunt mother. He nearly tripped over the doctor who was coming around the curtain. Max stumbled to catch himself and turned and nearly ran out of the ER. His world was closing in on him, his chest squeezed his heart with a death grip and he could barely breathe. Up the long hallway to the right, he saw a strangely colored light spilling out on the tile floor. It was coming from the doorway of the hospital chapel. He darted inside and found it empty. Inside he paced up and down the aisle between two small rows of pews. Eventually he slowed his pace until he was standing looking at the front of the chapel at a large crucifix with a very dead looking Jesus on it. He slipped into a pew and sat with his hands in his lap imitating devoutness. *I'm a chameleon.* Max thought. *I can do this.* Just as he was distracting himself with this little game of What does a person of faith look like? A man came from the doorway of small room off the side of the chapel. He was dressed in a black robe down to his ankles, his white socks making little rings just above his worn brown shoes. *Tacky.* Max thought, *I'd do a better job playing his role. With black trouser socks and a nice pair of loafers.* He looked him over again as the man lit a few candles and turned to face him. Max was struck with the kindness in his eyes and immediately felt bad for measuring him up.

"You a priest?" Max said as the man approached him.

"The collar give me away?" The man chuckled and sat sideways in the pew in front of Max, facing him with a hand extended. "Brother Lawrence," the man said warmly, "second year seminarian."

Max was quiet and so was Brother Lawrence. The silence wasn't awkward to either of them. Max looked down at his feet, sighed and looked again at the cross.

"Not sure how *that's* considered a Savior," Max said dryly. "Looks a little defeated to me."

"No offense," Brother Lawrence looked over his shoulder at the cross, and then back at Max, "but so do you."

Max looked around to be sure they were alone. "I'm at a loss," he began. "I met this woman about six years ago, when I was here in Chicago on business. She was completely captivating and coming on strong. I knew I shouldn't, but I'm not real good at denying myself any pleasure. Next thing I know, I'm in her bed and she's taking me out of this world…uh…sorry brother, no offense."

"None taken. Go on."

"Well, that was all it was, and then a few months ago, she reaches out to me. Says she saw in the paper that we …my dad and I…would be in Chicago for a ribbon cutting ceremony on a project we've completed. She wants to see me. I hem and haw and try to weasel out, but she's insisting it's important. So I set up a lunch meeting and when she shows up, she's emaciated like a walking skeleton. Scared the hell out of me. Says she's dying. Pancreatic cancer. I excuse myself to the bathroom and sneak out the door."

Brother Lawrence didn't react. He just sat quietly, kindly waiting for Max to continue.

"So then, last night, she shows up at our gala in a sequin gown and collapses after making it up the flight of stairs. I follow the ambulance to the hospital and sit waiting and wondering what to do, when finally her sister shows up with a little kid and Clarissa manages to tell me the little girl is mine!" Max's hands were shaking now and his voice trembling. He gripped the pew with both hands and tried to keep from falling apart. "Jesus, I'm a coward."

"Did you say you're married?" Brother Lawrence spoke in a low voice as if to say *your secret is safe with me.*

"Yeah. I'm married to a wonderful woman and we have six kids. Beautiful babies. And it's all falling apart, brother. It's all coming unglued. My father and I are dissolving our partnership. We make each other crazy. My wife is wondering what's up financially, and why I'm hardly home anymore. And this woman up the hall here is about to go home to Jesus," he makes a gesture nodding to the front of the chapel, "and I can't add that little brown beauty to the mix. I can't take care of her. Why the hell did Clarissa wait until she's nearly dead to tell me?"

Max gripped the pew tighter, white knuckling to hold back his tears. His lip began to quiver and his chest was tight again. He put his forehead on his hands to hide his face and shook with quiet sobs. Brother Lawrence put a hand on Max's shoulder and prayed silently for the peace and presence of God to come. Eventually, he calmed down and when he lifted his head, Lawrence handed him a box of Kleenex. Max wiped his face and leaned back in the pew. He looked up at the crucified one again and shook his head.

"I don't know what to do," he said finally. After a long pause, Brother Lawrence looked at him and said,

"One word for you?"

Max nodded, appreciative of any advice.

"The truth will set you free."

Max kept nodding and although he was terrified and ashamed of his circumstances, and had no faith that things would be okay, he continued to sit and nod and bask in just a little bit of peace.

Chapter 11

There was barely a congregation and Passover was only a week away.
Since Pastor Jacob was of the Messianic Jewish faith, he wanted to share
the meaning and traditions of a Passover meal with his new church. Denny
offered to host the Seder at her house. Her family and home was the
biggest, and she was looking forward to learning more about this new
holiday. She thought of the boy Jesus finding the matzah. And the man
Jesus hosting his last supper, the Passover he *"so desired to share with his
friends"*.

Pastor Jacob arrived with his wife, Jan and her four daughters, Lynn,
Ally, Kyle, and Jess. They were a boisterous bunch that reminded Denny
of the Loud family from Saturday Night Live. But she enjoyed them
immensely.

When Max was out of town, her household was mellow. She didn't
allow screaming. *"You'd better be bleeding or have a broken a bone if
you're screaming like that!"* Nor were they allowed to run around or
rough house indoors. When they were wound up, Denny would promptly
send them to bundle up and go outside and run off all of that hyperactivity.
This also doubled as exercise, she reasoned. She liked things mellow.

On the other hand, being around a big Italian family was a blast. The
energy, the fast talking, the laughter, the talking over top of each other, it
was all great fun, (as long as everyone went home after). Jan and Jacob's

family were breath of fresh air. Denny's kids paired off with Jan's kids and enjoyed them as well. They were fast friends.

For Passover, Denny pulled out the best linens and China and fabric napkins and her favorite crystal wine goblets and gold flatware. The kids had helped to press tablecloths and fold napkins into fans that stood upright on the dinner plates. Round tables were set up in the area between the dining and living room and covered with white linen table clothes for the kids to sit together. The handful of church attendants and Denny and Jacob and Jan and their assistant pastor, Dave, would sit at the formal dining table. Pastor and Jan arrived with loads of fancy olives, gourmet cheeses, breads and crackers along with some French Bordeaux and sparkling juice for the underage.

Dave wore his navy suit with the same tie and white shirt from the week before, or every week.

After Maxine and Helena laid out all the goodies on a cheese board, Jacob donned his religious clothing and stood at the head of the table and explained all the steps of the Passover meal. The younger kids congregated to listen and learn or got bored and went back to their seats to whisper and giggle and wait for the food. But the food didn't come. There were things on a Seder plate in the center of the table, herbs and horseradish and salt water, which they dipped with great ritual and ceremony. But no dinner. The cheese plate beckoned from the kitchen counter, but was well out of reach, and Denny frowned shaking her head in a slight jerky way when Alex made eyes and gestured toward it. Jacob did readings and formalities and most importantly, the telling of the story of the Jews' exodus from Egypt. Red wine was free flowing with several toasts:

Blessed are You, Lord, our God, King of the universe, who creates the fruit of the vine.

And later,

Blessed are You, God, our God, King of the universe, who has granted us life, sustained us, and enabled us to reach this occasion.

All were instructed to drink the cup of wine while seated, reclining on the left side as a sign of freedom.

The wine was a good distraction from the endless waiting for food. Eventually there were some dishes passed like gribenes, crispy onions and chicken skins that have been fried in schmaltz. And of course matzah bread that looks and tastes like cardboard. Denny was reminded of a comedian, Sabastian Maniscalco, who went to a Passover meal with his Jewish fiancé. In his standup routine, he made hysterical fun of the bad food and said the Italians should be in charge of the Passover. She couldn't have agreed more. *Where's the olive oil? The bread dip? When do we eat?*

The Passover meal was very satisfying for Denny. Although the food was not at all interesting, the rich significance and tradition made her feel closer to Jesus, the boy who grew up Jewish, with all the customs and feasts handed down from the book of the law. She was also growing closer to Pastor Jacob and his wife, Jan and their family. Jan's girls were all being home schooled, and they were free to get the kids together often. They bought a place on the Yukon River and Denny and the kids packed up and spent the day there often. In April they met in Swan Haven for the Celebration of Swans, when the thousands of trumpeter swans descend on their natural habitat. They made plans to attend the Adäka Cultural Festival in June with traditional and contemporary music, dance, drumming, storytelling, film screenings, daily artist demonstrations, art and traditional craft workshops, cultural presentations, an art gallery and more. Denny enjoyed the homeschooling freedom of living and learning.

Every day of life and all experiences were chalked up to schooling. If you can breathe you're still learning and all the world is your classroom.

In the early days of homeschooling, when Denny was less confident, she set up little desks in the den and ordered curriculum and had school hours, lunch time, and a routine that mimicked the school system she was familiar with. But soon the notepads and textbooks were making their way into the kitchen, the dining table, and kids were sprawled around the living room on couches and taking turns on the computer. As the years went by, the kids had bookshelves in their bedrooms, laptops and phones, and were busy coming and going on various hikes and outings. Whitehorse was a small town with a close-knit community. But there weren't many children around with the freedom to explore like Denny and Max's kids. So having another family in the area with boisterous lively healthy kids who weren't in school all day was an exciting change of pace for the family. When Max was home, he met Pastor Jacob and Jan, and enjoyed them very much. They were refreshingly different than the Whitehorse locals. Jacob had formidable knowledge in areas that Max was completely unfamiliar with, namely, the scriptures, and Jewish customs and traditions. Max found him interesting and appreciated that he didn't try to proselytize, but rather just discussed religion on an intellectual level. Denny, however, was far more interested in Jacob's missionary experiences. Jacob showed her pictures of his trips to Malawi where he met with other pastors and talked of open-air meetings and supernatural healings. "The people have so much more faith there. They have no choice. There is such poverty, and medicine is hard to come by. They must rely on God and His power. As soon as I would step off the plane and they understood why I was there, they would just crowd around wanting me to pray over them for healing. I was stunned. And I didn't really understand at first. My friend Bimba, who had invited me to come preach, said firmly, 'Lay your hands on them!' and when I did, things happened. Some fell over, some were healed. I was completely stunned. It was life changing."

Denny felt a ripple and thump across her taut belly and thought of Elizabeth's baby, John the Baptist, jumping in the womb at the greeting of Mary, her cousin, who was carrying baby Jesus. She chuckled thinking of the hunger she had to go and see these things for herself. She wanted to live the pages of scripture where miracles and signs and wonders were happening every day. And although some had said it was only Jesus that did those things, she read enough to see the signs and wonders all through the book of Acts, long after He was gone. And the Old Testament scriptures were full of signs and wonders and miracles as well. To Denny, this was the litmus test of religion. If these things were not happening, it was just man operating in his own wisdom. But if signs and wonders followed the preaching of the word, then God was with the people, His presence carried on the wings of the Word of God. The very God Himself showing Himself. This was what Denny longed for.

After Max had gone again, she spent more and more time with Pastor Jacob and his family. Winter was well underway in Whitehorse. The first snow fell in October and now it was November, and still no Max. Eventually, over some wine, they asked her about Max and his absences. She sighed and tried to explain, "Max and I have an unusual marriage. He can't seem to stay put for very long, and although he loves his family, he gets restless. It's difficult to watch. He goes from being jovial and charming and warm, to withdrawing completely into some dark place. He explained once that he cannot tolerate himself when he gets that way, and he certainly doesn't expect me to tolerate him. And off he goes. It used to be for a week or two here and there, home for a month or two, gone for a week. That sort of thing. But now, he's home four or five days, gone for two or three weeks. Before, it wasn't ideal. Now, it's become a problem."

"When was he home last?" Jacob said, "August?"

"Yes. That's when you met him." Denny lowered her voice to a whisper, "And I think there is someone else." Her eyes began to fill with tears, just as Alex came in from the deck.

"Are we staying for dinner?"

Denny looked lost and Jan spoke up for her, "I just made a huge salad and Jacob was about to cook steaks! How's that sound?" Alex ran back out the door shouting to the gang of kids,

"Yeah! We're staying!"

"Thank you," Denny squeezed the words from her throat, "you didn't have to do that. Are you sure?"

"Yeah, I'm sure!" Jan patted her knee and got up to go to the kitchen. She and Jacob made eye contact and she gave him a little nod.

"Why don't you take a little break," Jacob said to Denny. "Come with us to Hawaii. We're going on a business trip to discuss plans for a Bible college. Lynn is going with us, but she would have more fun with a roommate," Lynn was eighteen, Jen's oldest. Denny's head was spinning. She hadn't been away from her kids since she started having them sixteen years ago.

"I'm not sure a vacation is what I need at this point," she said hesitantly. She sounded very sad and Jacob and Jan both began talking at once.

"Look, Lynn will be bored to death. She doesn't need to be stuck in a room by herself. The room is already paid for. We have meetings planned. And we could also use your help with the ministry. You can get your feet wet and see if it's something you want to do more of."

"Jacob needs a lot more administrative help, and down the road, who knows? You may be going to Africa with us."

"It might do you good just to clear your head and get a little distance from everything"

"You'll have lots of time to soak up the sun and also do some work for the ministry. What do you say?"

Denny head was reeling. "When are you going?"

"Late next month. For ten days."

Denny was feeling wary, but hopeful. Maybe she could sort out what to do. Things with her marriage had become really heavy. For the first time in her life, she felt scared. She loved Max and had always fully trusted his care for her. He was an excellent provider. And he loved that she was home with his children. But lately, the bank account was not adding up. And Max had no straight answers for her. She began to wonder about making a living on her own. Would her whole world change? Did she need to go back to writing and editing full time? And what of the kids? Would they have to go back to school? Was it time to uproot the entire life she'd created so she could get a nine to five and not rely on anyone else? Seemed unrealistic with another baby on the way.

Denny loved Max very much. Bishop, a bouncy seven-year-old, Alex, now ten and inquisitive and intense, always ready to entertain. Maxine and Helena growing up too fast and ahead of their peers. At sixteen and fifteen, already enrolled in college and driving themselves more often than needing rides. Little people who needed her, but not in the all-consuming way an infant does. And the older siblings looked over the younger ones. Denny wasn't as certain about her place in the world. This unexpected pregnancy had thrown her for a loop. For the first time, a pregnancy seemed like a set-back. Inconvenient, at the very least. She caressed her near term belly, sighing. Ministry work is something she'd always wanted. But the kind of ministry she had in mind was not to be found in church. And traveling alone or with babies and children didn't sound ideal. She and Max hadn't had a serious heart-to-heart in far too long. She had begun to give up on any true partnership ventures with him. The Hawaii offer piqued her interest and she assured Jacob and Jan she would think it over. "Let's see how things go?" She looked down at her belly and shrugged. She was quiet during the ruckus of dinner with nine kids. Jacob and Jan nodded at her smiling gently.

Chapter 12

Max arrived late to the ribbon cutting ceremony. His father was midway through a speech about the health center and the city's collaboration with his firm. He thanked several contractors for a job well done and made a political plug for the mayor. Max approached and his father gave a pained introduction. Max was sure he would not have mentioned him at all if he hadn't shown up. He waved off his father with a humble gesture indicating he could keep right on. Max had no interest in speaking or acting this morning.

After the ribbon cutting and some handshaking and doughnuts and a brief tour of the building with the public, Max and his father parted ways. They had already established this would be their last project together. Max was putting together a team to start his own firm. As he was walking off toward his hotel, Bishop called out to him, "Maxwell!" Max turned and walked to meet his dad. "Where you off to? Let's get a drink. Celebrate." Bishop was brief, curt and authoritative. Max found it hard to say no to him. From the time he was a boy, this man was his hero. He would sweep into his life between projects and hoist him up on his shoulders and treat him like a prince. When Bishop was not home, Max read of his latest building accomplishments in the news, his face on the cover of Time, his projects on the covers of Architecture, Metropolis, and Blueprint magazines. He was famous. And Max was proud to be his son. But the pedestal his father was on was high and wobbly, structurally unsound with a weak foundation and building materials that were paper thin.

Bishop and Max's mom, Amber, divorced when Max was just eight. Max saw less and less of his father. And the pedestal he had built for him came crumbling down. He and his mother lived like they always had. Bishop wasn't around much when they were married. So in many ways, nothing changed. But Max was very hurt when his dad married again and began having kids with another woman. Kids who were his half siblings, but he never met. His dad sent plenty of money his way, but he rarely saw him. And when he did, he was a stranger. No longer hoisting Max on his shoulders and rough-housing and laughing with him. Instead he groomed him.

"One day you'll be in business with me, Son. Don't worry about football or hockey. You've got no time to be a jock. You need to stay focused on your studies," and he'd whip out a pencil and start diagraming his latest ideas. Max partly resented this, but he was secretly awed that his dad would invite him along on his journey when he was the most well-known architect in Canada. It made Max's heart race. But he couldn't let on. He was still angry after all. So he forced a bored look in his father's presence and studied his ass off in his absence. He devoured magazines, books, and classes on architecture. He mastered calculus, physics, engineering, and building technology, with painful diligence. The study times were laden with cranium-splitting frustration but art and design came effortlessly and he enjoyed them immensely.

His father was an unusual architect. He saw a project from the inside out, unfolding in a way that was unpredictable and unknowable. It was a collaborative with the client and all those who would be using the space. The vision would unfold in a roundtable way with everyone down to the janitor involved in the process. He saw it like an embryo in its development, beginning with the first cells that split and grow into a spinal structure and brain stem. No one really knew how it would develop, or what the finished details were. And the vision would flow like water, carving its way along and creating as it goes. His father was a spiritual man and wanted his creations to complement nature. Max on the other hand, had developed more of an industrial and technical view of architecture, yet he was deeply impressed with his father's work and appreciated his talent. He had even inherited some of his father's artistic vision and a love for his use of water and nature as a way to create harmonious structures. But Max was so different in his methods of planning and formulating the stages of a project, that the two of them were colliding endlessly. It was tiring, and after 25 years, Max thought it best to part ways. Over the years he had regained his respect for his father. And now that he was a man with a family, he also judged him less harshly. He knew what the call of creative work was like, how easy it was to be consumed with it and feel rewarded by it. The rewards were so immediate. So tangible. And the projects, however undetermined were still malleable and in the end, there was a sense of pride and accomplishment. Personal life didn't offer this comfort. Family life was fraught with questions of qualifications. Who am I to raise and influence these little people. I can only screw them up!

So Max had let his dad off the hook for his failed marriages. But he still resented him. It had become habit. It was a mixed bag of jealousy, envy, and the fear of becoming just like him. And now, he was in no mood to have a celebratory drink with him.

"How bout we meet for dinner?" Max was hoping his dad had a plane to catch and wouldn't be able to. But Bishop was jovial and smacked him on the shoulder.

"Perfect! Gibson's. Six 0'clock," As usual, Bishop called the shots.

"Sounds good," Max turned and walked away briskly toward his hotel, shaking his head. *Shit. How'd that happen.*

He arrived in his room in the early afternoon wishing he'd just had the drink with his dad. At least it would be out of the way, he wouldn't have to spend the afternoon dreading dinner. He took off his jacket and loafers and flopped on the bed with a sigh. Denny. He wanted to call Denny, but he couldn't bring himself to do it. She would sense something was wrong. More wrong than usual. He would wait and speak with her in person.

He opened his laptop and looked over his finances. It was bleak. He had no immediate prospects for work. The funds were leaking like water from a broken line. But he made a transfer after a little rearranging. Borrowing from the future to add funds to Denny's household budget. She was starting to worry. And he couldn't keep making excuses.

He closed his computer and thought of Clarissa and the child. He had left in a rush but returned after some time in the chapel. The gray-haired woman as it turns out, was not Clarissa's sister at all. She was a neighbor who noticed the girl was left alone in her apartment far too often. Rather than call the police, she invited Clarissa over and tried to befriend her to see if she could help. Clarissa seemed very wary of strangers and guarded, especially with her daughter. Clarissa was blameless when she was home with Jada. She didn't do drugs, she didn't drink, she never brought a man home. She felt better about leaving Jada alone than having a caregiver. Jada was a smart girl, and she would follow all the rules, not answering the phone or door, never leaving the apartment, keeping the volume low on the television. She had a phone but could only use it to play games or text with her mom or call in an emergency.

But in a short time, Dot had broken down her defenses and Jada had a new caregiver. She would come after school, and often stay nights when her mum was out. Once Dot won her over, Clarissa regretted the isolation Jada had lived in and was grateful for the help. Dot was a warm and wonderful gramma type for Jada, taking her on trips to the playground or shopping for school clothes. But more than outings was the warmth of

Dot's apartment. It was filled with decorations at every holiday. Jada loved the little Christmas, Thanksgiving, Halloween and Easter dish towels, and they did dishes together in the kitchen and Jada helped dry them and put them away. After dinner they watched game shows every night and Dot taught Jada how to crochet. Every Friday they made homemade pizza dough and Jada selected toppings. Mostly it was pepperoni and pineapple, but once in a while, Jada could be persuaded to try something a little different, like a Greek pizza, or spinach and feta, or garlic white pizza. Dot enjoyed taking care of her very much. But she was very worried since Clarissa had become sick. She knew she couldn't keep Jada full time. She was seventy-one. And although she could pass for sixty, because she had taken good care of herself physically, she didn't feel strong enough to take on parenting this poor thing alone.

Max and Dot talked briefly in the hallway outside the room where Jada clung to her vanishing mother.

"I just need a little time," Max was wincing and wringing his hands, trying to keep them from trembling.

"I don't have to tell you," Dot said whispering and pursed her lips like she didn't want to say it, "there is no time." Her eyes filled with tears and she looked away, steadying herself. "You weren't told about her, so the past is not relevant. But she is your responsibility." Dot was scolding him in a whisper that reminded him of his own mother. She began to tremble, "I cannot…"

"I know," Max interrupted. "I know." He took Dot's information and promised to be in touch. He couldn't bear to actually meet the little girl that was in the hospital bed with her mother. Not like this.

Chapter 13

Max arrived at Gibson's fifteen minutes early and ordered a scotch. He finished it before his dad arrived and ordered a second. The shaking in his hands settled down and he looked over the menu. When his dad arrived, he was dressed in a jacket and sweater, no tie, and dark slim jeans. Max grinned a little bit at his dad's look. He was always a well-dressed man, small and thin with impeccable posture. His clothes were trim and form fitting. Never anything sloppy or baggy. He carried himself far more rigid than his works would suggest. Where they were fluid and indefinite, his manner was concrete. Max stood to greet him, and his dad caught him off guard with a firm brisk hug and more patting on the back.

"We did it again, Son!" He was out of breath from the brisk chilly walk to the restaurant, but full of enthusiasm. "Another Belanger success! What are we having?" He looked from Max's glass to the approaching waitress,

"Scotch," Max's tone unenthused in contrast to his dad's.

"I'll have the same! And bring us a bottle of your best champagne." Bishop sat down across from Max and smiled. Max studied him. *It's like he doesn't know we're finished. Like this wasn't our last project. Why isn't he down?*

They ate warm crusty bread and appetizers of mussels and scallops bathing in a garlicky butter sauce, lobster cocktail, and the Chicago-cut prime angus steaks.

After a while, Max forgot about his troubles and bathed in the warm glow of the scotch and champagne and excellent food. He became relaxed and open and full of appreciation. His father would generously pick up the tab, as he always did, and when they were not locking horns over a building project, they actually enjoyed each other.

Bishop looked at his grown son and wondered where the time had gone. He remembered the way the kid had looked up to him. It was incredible and awkward. He knew he wasn't worthy of all that adoration. Once he and Max's mother had split, everything changed. The entirety of his fatherhood was based on getting Max to trust him again. To regain his friendship. He didn't care so much that Max wasn't in awe of him anymore. But he missed the friendship. And he'd tried to build rapport with him ever since. Max looked almost happy at the moment, and warm with a buzz, so Bishop threw out a line,

"You know, you can talk to me Son. I'm here to help you navigate a bit. I've learned a few things and gained a little wisdom over the years. And what's the sense in having a dad if you can't employ his services now and then?"

Max chuckled, "I'm pretty sure I've employed your services, Dad. We've worked together for 25 years!"

"Yeah, there's that. But the architect work isn't what I'm talking about. I'm talking about your family."

Max bristled visibly at the idea of his father advising him on matrimony or parenting. Bishop raised both hands in surrender, "No, no. Wait. Listen to what I'm saying. I've learned a lot from what I did *wrong*, Max. Don't think I don't know where I failed. I'm just saying I don't want you to make the same mistakes I have. And I'm here to help. That's all."

Bishop leaned back in his seat, arms still up like Max was pointing a loaded gun at him.

"Dad, put your hands down," Max shook his head and spoke softly. "I've got a lot on my plate right now. And…"

"I know you do. I'm here to help, Max. Any way I can."

Max sighed deeply and leaned back in his chair, thankful that the waitress had appeared to clear away some dishes and offer desert. "None for me, thanks," Max put his hands on his belly.

"How about a bottle of port to finish us up?" Bishop said to the waitress. As she left the table, he looked at Max and shrugged, "No one is driving," he said mischievously. "Now. Tell me about the waif on the floor at our cocktail party. And your sudden departure with the ambulance."

Max leaned in, elbows on the table, and ran his fingers through his hair as he rubbed his head. "She's the mother of a daughter I just found out about."

Bishop didn't respond. He just nodded slowly. "How old is the girl," he said finally.

"She's six? Eight? I can't remember. When were we first considering this Health Center Project?"

"You know," Bishop's face suddenly registered recognition. "Six. I think it was six years ago," he said. "The woman with the mayor. She was a beauty. I remember. Colombian was she?"

"Jamaican."

"Ahh. Yes. Well."

The waitress returned with their port and a couple small glasses. "Take as long as you like, gentleman. And congratulations on your project."

"How'd she know about that," Bishop said as she walked away.

"I told her. Gotta keep our name out there," he raised a glass to toast the project finally. Bishop held up his port.

"To the angry boy who became a brilliant man that I'm very proud of,"

"To overcoming projects that tried to kill us." Max said sarcastically.

"To family," Bishop said quietly. Max gulped down his port and poured another.

"I'm afraid I'm blowing it all, Dad," he whispered, starting to shake again.

"You're not gonna blow it, Son. What can I do to help?"

"I don't know. Maybe we could rethink this business. The firm. The way we work and fight together. I really thought we just needed to separate. But I'm not sure I can afford to right now."

"You know I always anticipated leaving the company to you, putting you in charge,"

"Yeah, but you can't do that while you're at the helm.

And you're not going to retire or kick off any time soon," they both chuckled at Max's boldness.

"Let's take a step back now that this project is finished. We can regroup. The idea of splitting up the company and going our separate ways never appealed to me. But, like you, I am tired of the friction between us on the job. Let's give it some more thought. In the meantime, the proceeds from this job should help for the time being." Bishop munched on some bread that was left on the table, took a swig of port. "Well, are you still involved with the Jamaican beauty or what?" Max was fiddling with his phone.

"She's dead," he said as he tossed his phone across the table for his father to read the text. It was from Dot: Clarissa just passed away quietly. I'll be taking Jada to my place. She could really use some family. Please don't wait long.

"Jesus." Bishop sat and looked at his son. Neither of them spoke for a long time.

Chapter 14

Max sat watching Dot stir her tea in slow deliberate circles. The table against the wall, with two small cane chairs, only had room for two. A bright linen tablecloth covered in purple and white wisteria vines draped the table, the wood framed chairs painted lavender and white checked to match. To Max, everything seemed miniature in this room. And everything matched. From the patterned dessert plates to the cup and saucer in front of Dot, to the glass she had given him filled with ice water. The purple blossoms were everywhere, dangling like grapes from the wallpaper to the dish towels, to the glassware and napkins and throw rugs. He sat watching her thinking this might be the worst poker game of his life. The stakes were too high. It was certainly no fun. The pitiful little kid in the living room sat in front of the television. Her coat neatly folded and sitting next to her, a small suitcase packed and waiting behind the couch. Max watched as Dot stopped stirring, picked up the teabag, wrapping the string round and round the spoon and pressing the tag with her thumb, squeezing the tea from the bag. As the last drops landed in the cup, Max's mind was whirling. *I can't. I don't know... I don't know what to do. I need some time. What the hell. I don't know what to do.* Dot set the spoon down on the saucer with a determined click. It was his move. She wasn't bluffing. She waited. Finally, Max had an idea. He jumped up, put his glass in the sink, and said, "Alright," and walked through the living room to the door of the apartment. Dot followed and stood in front of Jada, blocking the tv. "It's time, honey," she spoke tenderly. Jada got up, clicked off the show she was watching and picked up her wool coat. Her mother had bought her the velvet trimmed navy wool coat with big wooden buttons down the front and pleats in the back after she had seen Miracle on 34th Street. She decided her little Jamaican needed to look fashionable in the Chicago climate. She wore a pink corduroy shift to the knees over a long-sleeved white blouse with pressed peasant collar. Her blue wool cable knit knee socks matched the coat perfectly. And the black suede ankle boots were only worn on special occasions. Jada put on her coat and grabbed her Cossack hat and gloves, picked up her suitcase and followed Max. Her heart was pounding but she was using all of her strength to be brave, and not cry or make a fuss. Max opened the door, and Dot squatted low to look into Jada's face. "Now you remember what I promised. Right? We will be in touch. And we will see each other again." Jada's eyes were welling up with tears and she threw herself into Dot, nearly knocking her off balance. Her little arms didn't fit around Dots middle, but she buried her head in her bosom and squeezed Dot with all of her might. Then she broke away and swallowed hard.

Her mother had whispered many things to her as she slipped in and out of consciousness in her hospital bed. You will have a big fambly in Canada. You will have a Daadie now. Max is a good man. He will take care of you. Be brave my Jada, my gift from God. Max nodded at Dot. "I'll be in touch." And he held out his hand for the little girl. They silently made their way to the elevator, and when Max heard the apartment door close behind them, he shuddered.

Oh God. What have I done.

In the elevator, Max looked down at Jada and said, "Where do you like to eat in the city?" She lit up and cried out "Dr. Bird's! Oh my mum and I go whenever there is a birthday or a special occasion. I love it."

"Well, this is a very special occasion. A sad and special occasion. So how about we go there, and I will invite your grandfather! You can tell us what to eat."

"I have a grandfatha?"

"You do! His name is Bishop Belanger"

"Oh my." Jada noticed Max's hand was a little shaky. His forearm was strong and muscular, with soft brown hair. And he smelled good.

Max managed to reach his father in the cab ride to Dr. Bird's. Relieved that he hadn't left Chicago yet, he nearly cried when Bishop agreed to head over and meet him. The restaurant was a quaint little place more for carry out than eat in, but the industrial tables and painted metal chairs and bright colors gave it a fun feel. A stainless-steel bar with the front covered with varnished wood pallets, map covered walls, and a vintage neon light of a red bellied streamer tail, Jamaica's own national bird, thus called Doctor Bird's.

"Spicy beef patty with cheese and curry fries," Jada was saying as soon as they walked in. They found a booth and had the place to themselves, as it was too late for lunch, and too early for dinner. Max went and put in their order while Jada and Bishop visited. Max looked over and wondered how it was possible he had just watched this little girl at her mother's funeral. She was chatting happily and seemed to love Bishop immediately. But only that morning he had watched her stand like a perfect statue, holding the hand of Dot and looking at her mother's simple pine box coffin. Dot had arranged a burial before Clarissa had died. There was no one to call. Her family back home in Jamaica had not spoken with her since she left as a teenager. There was no one at the burial except Jada, Dot, and the pastor who did the most minimal reading and service he had ever witnessed. The only flowers were the ones Max picked up, nearly an afterthought on his way there. He placed the bundle of cala lilies on her casket and looked at the ground until it was over, about ten minutes. And then they met at Dot's apartment after.

He watched his father and Jada. One would think they'd known each other for years. He brought the patties over and the three of them munched and enjoyed the Jamaican tunes, the men lauding Jada for her good taste and excellent dining selection. But Max was still quite nervous and restless. When Jada went off to the restroom as if she owned the place, Max quickly blurted out to his father, "I gotta ask you for a huge favor, Dad. Just a few days. I can't take her to Whitehorse. I haven't even talked to Denny. I can't do that over the phone. I gotta see her in person. I can't take her with me to do that. Can you keep her? Just for a few days? Or even one day. A few hours? Something," He was whispering and rambling without taking a breath trying to get it all out before Jada returned. His hands were shaking and his voice desperate. But Bishop was calm and serene and just reached out and patted Max's hand. "It's okay, Son. It'll be fine. She'll be fine. And yes. I can keep her while you go talk to Denny."

Max was still rambling, "I mean, I don't know what Denny will do. I don't know what the kids will think. I don't know…"

"I know. It's okay. It's okay Max." Bishop was grateful that he could help, and that his son actually asked for his help. When Jada approached, Max leaned back against the padded booth and sighed deeply. He wasn't so sure it was okay. Or that anything would ever be okay again.

"Whaddya say you stay with me and let your dad fly home to his big family. And then you and I can go surprise them in a day or two?" Bishop was smiling warmly at her like they had a secret. And for some reason, Jada felt herself warming up to him much quicker than Max. Grandfatha Bishop. Yes. This could be fun.

"Would that be ok, Max?" Jada looked at him not sure he would approve. Max played along like he didn't know.

"Well, I suppose it would give me some time to prepare a place for you and talk to my wife and kids about you. And your grandfather doesn't often see us in Canada, so it would give you a little more time with him. I don't know. Would you like that?" Max was frowning and looking like he was trying to decide what was best for her. He was talking to her like she was his, shifting over into parenting role. And it felt quite natural. Jada was nodding like it was fine with her. She looked a bit relieved that she would be staying with Bishop. And so it was settled. Max would fly back to Canada tonight. And Bishop would follow shortly with Jada. When Bishop returned to his hotel room with his newest granddaughter, he decided they would not stay there. He thought of all she had just lost and said goodbye to, and staying in her own city of Chicago in a hotel on this particular night did not sit right with him. It was too depressing. No. He must take her now, somewhere. And hope Max didn't drag his feet making arrangements.

"Have you ever been on an airplane?" Bishop asked Jada as he packed up his garment bag and his toiletries. She was looking through some magazines marveling at the unusual buildings her new friend Bishop Grandfatha had designed, while he was putting the last of his belongings in his luggage. He noticed her little suitcase resembled something from an antique store. Retro and cute, yes. But it had seen better days.

"I was thinking, if you would like, we could go to Niagara Falls on the way to Whitehorse. We could stop off at the mall first and do a little shopping. Would you like that?"

"Oh yes. I would! I think I would love to see an airplane and see Niagara Falls."

"Well, little one, you're not just going to see an airplane! We will fly in one!" Bishop called his pilot/driver to inform him of the plan: Come retrieve us at Bloomingdales in two hours. Flying to Niagara District Airport later this evening, a light dinner on the plane for two, and accommodations at the Falls upon arrival. Jada seemed comfortable and still surprisingly cheerful considering her circumstances. The activities were keeping her distracted and every waking hour was full of new experiences.

Bloomingdales was bustling with holiday merriment and although shopping was not Bishop's favorite thing to do, having Jada with him made it much more interesting. She was pointing in every direction and wide eyed and completely awed by the 50-foot Christmas tree. As Bishop watched the magic in her eyes his heart ached for her. This Christmas she would be without her mother. *Max, I hope you know what you're doing. And for her sake, I sure hope this works.* He sighed and returned his attention to Jada. "Let's go find you some luggage," he smiled and she followed him, her hand in his through the lights and glimmer of retail. He didn't want to tire her after all she had been through already, and he was quite surprised she wasn't breaking down, or tantruming, or collapsing with exhaustion. Instead, she immediately fell in love with a pearl pink Aviator bag on wheels and asked if she was allowed to pull it through the store. The color matched her shift perfectly, and Bishop was impressed with her selection. He paid for the bag and slipped her little suitcase inside it for the time being, extended the handle and tipped the bag offering it to her. "Madam," She pulled it proudly through the store to their waiting car out front. Bishop's driver put the bag in the trunk, and she and her grandfather reclined in the back seat where she promptly fell asleep.

Chapter 15

Bishop was becoming a little nervous. The child had fallen asleep in the car ride to the airport and remained asleep when they arrived. He scooped her out and carried her in his arms up the airstairs of the leased jet and settled her gently onto the divan and covered her. She never made a peep. He was afraid if she woke during take-off, or slept too long, she may wake disoriented and upset. But he took his chances, thinking the poor child needs all the sleep she can get. Surprisingly, take-off was uneventful, she snoozed away like a sleeping beauty, and Bishop settled in and worked on a crossword puzzle a while. The flight attendant brought him a hot mug of cappuccino with croissants.

"Any possibility there's hot cocoa for Jada when she wakes? And she will probably be hungry. So we'll have dinner shortly. The mini meatballs, the cheeseboard, and some more of these croissants. These are delicious!"

"Yes. I think I can finagle some hot chocolate, sir. Can I get you anything else?"

"No, this is fantastic. Thanks so much."

In a short time the cabin was filling with the smell of hot meatballs and warmed croissants. Jada stirred, and Bishop, who was keeping a hawk eye on her where she slept, held his breath. She looked around, rubbing her eyes sleepily. The cabin was dark but for dim overhead lighting in long strips above. Soon, her eyes adjusted to the light. She turned saw

Bishop sitting in his chair under a reading light. She squinted at him as
though he were familiar, like she was trying to place him, and suddenly,
she smiled and said, "Grandfatha! Are we flying?"

Bishop relieved, let out his breath and sighed happily. Thank God. He
couldn't believe how adaptable this kid could be. He adored her to the
moon and back, and he'd only know her since lunch. She got off the divan
and came to sit next to him. He made room, moved his snacks and
crossword, and invited her on his lap. She snuggled into him and he
thought she might go back to sleep. But then the flight attendant was back
with steaming hot cocoa and warm things to eat and Jada lit up again. She
was clearly hungry and ate two whole croissants before her cocoa had
cooled enough to sip, and she desperately wanted to sample those
meatballs, but they too were piping hot. She started gabbing about all the
things around her, from the dark windows to the sky outdoors, the little
lights on the plane's wings, to the strange little fans above Bishop's seat
that he turned on and off and toward her and away from her since she
could not reach them and he couldn't have her standing on the seat, or
him. The flight attendant returned, took away their plates and cleared
space for dessert. Bishop sipped his cappuccino while a very grown-up
acting Jada sipped her cocoa in unison.

"Cheesecake! My favorite!" Jada said as it was served in front of her.
For a moment, a sad look came across her face.

"What is it, sweetie?" Bishop looked into her eyes, a finger under her
quivering chin.

"It's my mum's favorite, too." Her eyes filled with tears, but she
wouldn't let a single one drop. She looked up at the ceiling, blinking and
sniffing, like she was trying to keep it together.

"Honey, it's okay to cry. You love your mum very much. It's okay to
be sad." But she turned away and looked out the window. When she

turned back to him she had regained her composure and was again acting like a little adult.

"My mum told me that Max, er Fatha has lots of kids already. Is that right?"

"Why yes it is, Jada."

"And I will live with them?"

Bishop tapped his foot nervously. Oh boy. Uh, yeah. Sure! I think so. But I don't want to make any promises. If push comes to shove, I may have to keep you myself. God help us if Denny doesn't!

"We're going to go there soon. Just after our little side trip to Niagara Falls. Do you remember that we were going to see the falls?" Just then they were told to prepare for descent and landing. "See? We'll get some more sleep, and then tomorrow we'll go see the falls. How's that sound?"

"You're not sure if they'll want me are you Grandfatha?"

"Oh, no. No, Jada. Don't talk like that. It's all going to work out. I promise. YOU, my dear, will be just fine. Everything is going to be just fine, okay?" Jada nodded slowly, a little skeptical. She had to believe him, though. What choice did she have. He was her new Grandfatha Bishop. He wouldn't lie to her. Would he?

Chapter 16

Goldenrod Belanger lay quietly on her side in the king bed of her log home's master suite. The sun would not be rising much before noon, as darkness in Whitehorse creeps in by October and doesn't start to creep out until February, and it was now mid-December. The snow that falls in early October never melts away but hides beneath newer snow which continues in layers accumulating for the entire season until it has blanketed every house, tree, and roadway. Denny was awakened by the cautionary back-up sounds from huge snow removal trucks, their bright headlights reflecting off the white snow against a pitch-black night depicting a strange landscape from some uninhabited planet. The loader and dump truck had arrived just as she felt a pop and gush of release from between her thighs, accompanied by a strong vice-like contraction. There was no returning to sleep.

Denny was 41 years old and 42 weeks pregnant with her sixth baby, three of which were sprawled out around the king bed with her, sleeping soundly. When her contraction subsided, she quietly snuck out of the bed, retrieving a towel from the floor and holding it between her legs, and made her way to the bathroom. Her mother, Helen was in the next room. She had arrived just a few days shy of Denny's due date. With her experiences with Denny's previous births, she suspected the baby would not come much before forty weeks. All five of her other children, with the exception of little Amber, came between forty-two and forty-three weeks. The oven is a slow cooker, they would joke. Only Amber came a little "early" at thirty-nine and a half weeks. Denny sat on the toilet and arranged her day in her head. She was relieved to be in labor. Although she didn't mind pregnancy, the last couple weeks were always the worst. The inability to get comfortable, the pressing on the lungs, the feeling there's not enough room to breathe properly, leaning and arching back to elongate the torso, the heartburn, the burning sensation from a bony heel of her baby pressing so hard from within, that Denny wondered if the muscle tissue just below her rib had a hole in it, and she dreamed the foot popped through her side.

She smelled the coffee brewing which she prepared the night before and had on a timer. She was careful not to wake anyone, esteeming her alone time and her time with God. She could hear Helen stirring. She ran through the checklist in her head. She would go into her closet where there was a small lamp, candles, incense, essential oils, her Bible and other devotionals. She took her coffee daily in the closet and studied the scriptures and prayed. Eventually she heard the kids stirring, and she made her way out to the kitchen to greet them. As they sat for pancakes, Helen smiled at her daughter. "How long?" she said with a knowing grin.

"I've been up a couple hours. Water broke. I'm probably at about three or four." Centimeters that is. Helen offered to rub her shoulders, her back, or draw a bath.

"Just let me know if I can do anything, okay?"

Being midwife to Denny was exciting. But it was also tricky. Denny was supremely independent and was not comforted by a lot of touch or fuss. She was like a mother cat who needed to go hide in a dark place with no disturbances or interruptions. When it was time, she would go off by herself and get down to the business of birthing. At this stage, she was happily taking care of breakfast, setting the kids on the course for their day, and pausing for long intervals of strong contractions. Maxine and Helena were heading out to the local Yukon University where they were enrolled part time. Amber, Alex and Bishop had planned to go to the library with Nana Helen, but the day would be rearranged now. As much as Denny wouldn't mind being left completely alone, Helen wouldn't have it. She asked the kids what they would be working on, helped them tidy their rooms and then suggested they bake some goodies to have on hand for the rest of the day. Alex and Bishop helped plan the menu. The excitement was tangible. The older girls hesitated, not sure if they should go to class if their mom was going to deliver today, but Helen assured them they would only be waiting around for the big event. Denny went into her master bathroom, passing by the bed where she discovered Amber just waking up. Denny sat down and caressed her hair and kissed her on the cheek. "You plan to get up today, sleepy head?" Amber sat up and looked at her mom's face as it started to go blank, her eyes far away and her breathing changing, slowing down, deliberate long breaths. Amber smiled, "Today's the day, mom!"

When the contraction was over, Denny sat still on the bed recovering, while Amber went and started the bath for her. She didn't say a word, but her mom went in and shut the door. Amber tore the sheets off the big bed and retrieved the plastic to cover the mattress, then threw down soft cotton blankets, then the fitted sheets, then the folded middle sheet, then she ripped open a package of chux and set it by the bed. She plugged in an electric throw for Denny to use in the bed or in the chair, which she also covered with plastic and sheets and chux. Birth was an exciting time for Amber. She remembered Bishop's birth with awe when she was only five. She had hoped there would be many more in the house, but Denny had a long lapse after Bishop. Everyone assumed the family of five was complete, until little Joe came along, quite unexpectedly.

Denny had long ago given up on her eight babies. It was becoming too lonely to raise them on her own. Her love for Max was strong, but the reality was, they lived separate lives. She had also discovered the teen years were more demanding than toddlers ever were. And more expensive also. The home needed repairs, the kids wanted vehicles, the grocery bills were higher, the marriage was full of holes. And Denny felt like she'd been wrestling long enough and wanted to tap out. She stepped into the warm bath and shouted out a thank you to her Amber.

"Just call if you need me, mom. Everything is all set up," Amber spoke through the closed door, and went to find Helen and get some breakfast. She skipped through the house excited. Helen smiled at her, "Ah, my midwife apprentice! It's a wonderful time isn't it?" Nana Helen served up a healthy stack of pancakes for Amber and poured her a mug of steaming tea. "I just love it," Amber said. "I think I should come live with you and learn all about birth and babies!"

"Ahh, honey. That's a lovely thought, but I'm rarely catching babies anymore unless they're your siblings! I can certainly direct you along the path, though. You can get plenty of study in between now and when you're old enough to really apprentice."

Amber wanted to ask a million questions about all the births Nana Helen had attended, but she stopped herself. With her own mother laboring in the next room, she didn't want to think on any precarious stories or unhappy endings. She knew they happened, however. Amber had wisdom beyond her dozen years. She had a solid dependable bearing and was like a kid at the beach unafraid of the surf that batters and rolls and pounds in and out with unceasing boldness. She stands watchful. And unafraid. Yet not aloof or unmoved. Just strong. Accepting. And incredibly mature. Bishop and Alex began mashing bananas for banana bread, while Helen cleaned up the last of the breakfast dishes, listening carefully for any signs of Denny calling out for her. She would nod at

Amber occasionally who would run and put an ear to the bathroom door and come back shaking her head. When the bread was done, Helen checked on Denny with a warm slice, "Need something to eat, hon?" Denny had moved to the bed and was lying quietly in the dark. She took the bread but barely acknowledged Helen. She was quiet and still. Helen watched her for a few minutes. Quietly checked the baby's heart rate, asked if she could get her anything, made sure her water was full by the nightstand. And left her alone. "Won't be long now," she told Amber. "Let's get the stroganoff on so we don't have to do that later." Bishop, Alex and Amber all cut up mushrooms and onions while Helen seared the beef cubes and added them all to a big pot, covered with homemade vegetable and tomato juice and let the meat simmer. Maxine and Helena would be home from their classes anytime. Helen began to have the familiar feelings of fear and uncertainty that comes with any birth. The moments when you wonder if everything is okay. If the baby will come okay. If the mother will have complications. If the magical beautiful moment will turn into a tragedy, an emergency, a trauma. No. None of that. We don't allow fear. Risk is a reality. But fear is of no use. And simultaneously, the girls arrived from school as Denny let out a loud groan from the bedroom. Helen went to the door and paused until she heard her daughter, "Mom! Mom!" and she burst into the room to find her laying on her side holding a knee to her chest and there between the sheets lay a squirming baby boy, a little on the gray side. Denny was smiling and slightly hysterical with the surge of oxytocin. Helen got to work wrapping and wiping down little Joe, bringing color to his little body and planting him in Denny's arms after she scooted up in the bed. Helen covered mom and baby with the electric blanket and Amber and the other kids all rushed in, tucking pillows behind her back and bringing her more banana bread and water and anything else she might want. A hush came over the room full of girls as they stared at little Joe. He was beautiful, and black as the night.

Chapter 17

Max arrived just in time to see his oldest daughters walking in the house. The twins that weren't twins. Both had grown more than he could comprehend. Both with long slender legs and long blonde hair like Denny's. He almost couldn't tell them apart but for the spring in Helena's step whereas Maxine carried herself with more of a steady stride that said *I'm responsible. I'm the firstborn. I'm in charge here.*

They were in the house and out of sight, oblivious to the cab that let him out right behind them. They were chatty and excited and quite unaware of their surroundings. Once inside, Max felt a peculiar emptiness in the living areas. He set down his bag and listened for voices. Bishop ran from the hallway that led to the master bedroom, bare feet slapping against the heated tile floor, she grabbed a root beer from the fridge and ran right past him to the bedroom again like he was invisible. She was a peanut of a child, tiny for her age, with the same long blonde hair as the others. At seven years old, she was the baby and the little darling of the entire family. *Put her down. Let her do it. She can walk.* These were all things Denny found herself repeating endlessly since the little peanut was born. She was irresistible and the "twins" as well as Amber and Alex doted over her endlessly. Whatever she pointed to, they would fetch for her. They finished her sentences for her with baby talk. They carried her everywhere. Denny was afraid Bishop would never walk, talk, or do a darned thing for herself with all the attention and affection that was showered on her. But eventually, however late, she did walk, and then she ran. She ran everywhere. Ran up and down the hallways of their log home, ran from the kitchen to the bathroom and back again. Always on the go, she made up for all that time she had spent on her little queen throne. It's as if one day she hopped off and had not stopped since. But she was an easygoing and pleasant child. Her motor ran full speed morning till night, then, just as suddenly, she fell asleep and zonked for a good nine hours. Max stood thinking on his little revved up baby girl and her boundless energy when he heard the unmistakable gurgling, high- pitched sound of a newborn. The sound pierced through his heart and brought tears to his eyes. He took off his shoes and made his way back to the master bedroom where the whole family was gathered.

Maxine and Helena scooted between the bed and the wall trying to get a better look at little Joe. They both stared wide eyed, mouths open. They looked at each other, made a face, and looked back at their mother. Denny was twirling tiny black curls of his hair between her fingers and looking in awe at her newest little one. Bishop and Alex were on the bed on hands and knees ogling the newborn, Helen stood over Denny and her eyes went from her daughter to little Joe and back to Denny, who never looked up. Just as Helen was about to clear the room so she could help check over Denny and the baby and deliver the afterbirth, Max appeared in the doorway. The kids all shrieked and ran to him, as he knelt down to embrace Bishop and Alex, and stood hugging Maxine and Helena, looking over their shoulder at Helen and Denny. Denny, without looking up, gently lifted a sheet over her newborn and covered him from view. She didn't return Max's gaze. Helen took the opportunity to shoo everyone, "Okay, I think Mommy needs a minute and I need to look her over. How about you all wait in the other room, and I'll call you when she and baby are all cleaned up and rested?"

Max was unusually quiet and humble, leading the kids out of the room, and assuming Helen would tell him if there was a problem. As soon as the door was closed, Helen tended to Denny. In no time, she gave birth to the placenta. Helen diligently examining it for any tears, or missing parts. It was complete and perfect. She looked over Denny's bottom. No tears, no stitches necessary. Her bleeding was heavy, but not alarmingly so. She changed the sheet and chux beneath her, and gently washed her up. Denny was quiet and cooperative. Her independence had given way to a shaky, tired, teary and receptive Denny. Helen moved swiftly and worked quietly. She examined the little boy and he was a perfect treasure, of a very different color. When she was finished, she returned little Joe to his mother and sat close.

"Apparently, I have some explaining to do." Denny said dryly.

In the family room, Bishop was asking no one in particular, "Why is the baby's skin so dark? And his hair?" Maxine and Helena looked at each other again and shrugged wide eyed and then quickly looked at their father, who was frowning. He hadn't really had a glimpse of the little guy yet. Alex piped up, "I think he's African." The "twins" frowned at her and shook their heads, Helena putting a finger to her lips to hush her. Max felt like he was in a twilight zone. His kids were growing up and where had he been? They are not the little toddlers he used to toss around and cook with and tumble around in the snow with. They were so grown up. Even little Bishop, at only seven was so articulate and clever. Where had he been? The universe had stopped suddenly and he was having an immense realization. He had missed so much. So very much. Too much. Waves of grief and regret threated to knock him to the floor right in front of his offspring. The guilt was creeping up from his gut to the back of his throat. Maxine, watching him, asked, "Dad. Are you okay?" She was old enough to know that the baby in her mother's bed could not belong to Max. And she began to seethe with anger at Denny. But Max just walked by her, dazed, and went to the bedroom. Helen guarded her daughter. She didn't know what was going on, but she knew Denny was in a very vulnerable position, having just given birth. She didn't want her upset or threatened in any way. But when she saw Max's demeanor, her guard relaxed. He looked broken and more than a little lost. She looked to Denny for direction. Denny nodded at her mother who rose and gently stroked Max on the back as she passed him and left the room, shutting the door behind her.

Denny uncovered her little bundle so Max could get a good look at him. His eyes widened and he sat stunned for a long time. And then he began to sob. He sat in front of little Joe and Denny and fell apart. Denny was moved but didn't know what to think. She waited quietly, assuming he was filled with grief that she had someone else's child.

Chapter 18

Denny loved flying and was thankful to have a window seat. She wore her baby in a carrier, nursing him on demand. Her excitement grew with the gust of the engines as the aircraft sped down the runway at takeoff and her heart lifted and lightened as they made their way through the clouds to their cruising altitude. Little Joe slept through the entire thing. Denny's facial muscles formed an involuntary smile. She had not felt herself smile in quite some time. As she gazed out the window with a more optimistic perspective, high above the clouds, the earth shrinking beneath her, she began to unpack the memories that brought her to her current circumstance:

Justin stood at the edge of a large gym mat; kids lined up to have a turn to speak with him. When Denny arrived and asked for him, a teenager behind the counter motioned to the line. He was six foot or more with the physique of an Olympic gymnast. Cut, carved and sculpted, but no resemblance to a body builder or weightlifter. He was the darkest black man Denny had ever seen. And he would be her instructor. She felt nervous and awkward as she stood in line to talk with him, nearly losing her nerve. She was close to running out. "This is a dumb idea. What was I thinking. I'll never be able to do this." But just as she turned to go, he was saying, "Denny? Are you Denny Belanger?" She sighed deeply and turned around to face him. His expression was very gentle, his eyes kind and inquisitive as he reached out a hand to greet her.

"Yes, we uh, spoke on the phone."

"Justin Keen. I'm glad you could make it. Let's go have a seat for a minute over there where we won't be interrupted," he motioned to a booth against the far wall near a small café' area she hadn't noticed before. He clapped his hands and sent the kids off to shower. Each bowed to him before turning away and running to the locker room. "Can I get you a coffee? Or a smoothie or anything from the snack bar? A water?"

"I'm fine thanks," Denny pointed to the bottle of green tea she had with her. "To be honest, I'm having second thoughts about all of this. I just don't know…"

"Why don't you start by telling me what happened if it's not too painful. You came here for help. And we're just talking. You don't have to decide anything. You don't have to do anything. Maybe let's just talk for a bit, yeah?"

He was very disarming. And she softened and worked up the nerve to tell him about the incident, her hands nervously playing with the cap on the tea bottle. "I was just loading my groceries into the Jeep. I was about to turn and shut the passenger door when I was grabbed by the hair and my face slammed into the back seat," her hands and voice were trembling. She didn't look at Justin. "I was pinned by the weight of this guy behind me and then his hand was over my mouth. Before I could even scream he was groping me." She stopped talking and twisted the cap off her tea and took a swig, trying to steady herself. When she looked up, his eyes were full of compassion and kindness. "Thank God our friend Bill showed up," She sighed deeply, visibly relieved.

"Bill?"

"He's a friend of the family. Works for the highway department. We've known him for years. Well, he just happened by, like a gift of God.

Shouted at the creep who was assaulting me and startled him. The guy ran off across the parking lot and Bill chased him for a little bit, but I think he worried about leaving me, and wanted to be sure I was okay. So he was back and the other guy was long gone."

"Did you go to the police?" Justin regretted he'd asked as soon as it was out of his mouth. He knew that wasn't the point. And it made no difference to her experience. "I'm sorry," he said quickly.

"No. Bill really wanted to call them immediately. And I was just too shook up. I just wanted to be home and feel safe. I was a coward."

"Woah. No. Come on, now. That's not true. You were seriously threatened and had every reason to be afraid."

Denny lifted her eyes slowly to make eye contact with Justin. "I used to be very different," she sighed heavily. "When I was in middle school I slammed a boy into his locker for groping me. I don't know what happened, but I feel like I've lost that person," her voice was low and weary, filled with defeat.

"I'd like to help you find her again." Justin said firmly. Denny nodded slowly as he continued, "Tuesdays and Thursdays. Six PM? I shouldn't need more than six weeks. I can give you tools and techniques that will help you. You'll be equipped to defend yourself and disable any threats. This training will also help you to heal from what happened to you."

Denny was skeptical. But his confidence was contagious. She looked around the room. In this gym, surrounded by punching bags, wrestling mats, teens wearing gis, and the slight scent of sweat in the air, it struck her just how frail and insecure she had become over the years since she married Max. And it made her angry. Within a month, she had tapped into that anger, and mixed it together with every unjust thing that had ever happened to her and came up with a cocktail of ferocious energy that both surprised and scared her. Add to that an unexpected chemistry had developed between them. Denny was not comfortable being vulnerable.

But angry, she could do. And Justin was rattling her cage. Over the years, he had trained in Jujutsu, Judo, mixed martial arts, and a little boxing. From the eastern practices, he had honed his character with the highest standards of integrity and self-mastery which Denny found terribly attractive. Justin was a securely married man. A consummate professional. Serious-minded. No nonsense. But for some reason, Denny's antics in their time together made him laugh out loud. She was not trying to penetrate his perfect composure. Quite the contrary, she was self-conscious and mostly embarrassed by the grappling, footwork, throws, sweeps and takedowns. She was as awkward as the pimply junior high kids that were in and out of the gym. And when she would dig deep to muster up a seriousness for their sparring, it would send Justin into an enormous struggle to stay focused and not laugh. Oh but he enjoyed her. And the talks they had after class over a protein drink or a smoothie were stirring some dangerous feelings in him. He was finding her irresistible and even considered ending their training for the fire that was building between them. She was constantly turning red, or catching her breath at his nearness, making concentration utterly impossible. She was eating up the physical contact and he knew it. She was starved for male closeness. Denny felt guilty as hell for the pleasure she received from his physical contact. It was a torturous mix of pleasure and guilt, anger and self-loathing, fear and excitement. On the drive home each night, she told herself to cut it out. She had already learned enough to lash out at a predator. She was confident she could defend herself against the worst of them. She didn't need any more of Justin's help. But he felt soooo good. The way they sparred together, the moves he put on her, the scent of him drove her mad. And then she'd get mad at Max.

Where the hell was Max? He was her husband. Why was she so alone? Max was offering her up on a silver platter with a little towel draped over his arm. Max could care less. And he'd left her wide open.

Chapter 19

On the long flight across the Pacific, Jacob and Jan were very attentive and kind. Jacob had been a pastor for many years and had an easy relaxed way of listening and gently eliciting confessions from Denny. She ended up telling him all kinds of personal things as the hours droned on. She shared more of her turbulent marital story, including the brief encounter with her self-defense trainer. The relationship ended promptly after one indiscretion, both of them disappointed in themselves. She never told Justin about her pregnancy. "Besides being unfaithful and weak, I am also a friggin coward and was never able to tell him I was pregnant. And the more time that went by, the easier it was not to tell. How can I condemn Max when I've done the same thing? I couldn't bear to meet his Jada. It's just a giant mess. And here I am flying away." Her lips pursed tightly together, her forehead furrowed, nostrils and jaw alternately flaring and clenching, Jacob patiently nodding and listening. Eventually, Jacob interrupted Denny's outflow of guilty ramblings, asking gently, "May I make a suggestion, Denny?"

"Of course," she paused her disjointed confession and took a breath.

"Perhaps you could treat yourself as if you're helping one of your children. Or a dear friend. We tend to be infinitely harder on ourselves than we are toward those we love." He paused smiling, eyebrows raised in a peace offering sort of way. "Give yourself a break. Some room. Take the club of self-beratement from your hand and just set it aside." Denny tossed her head against the back of her seat and chuckled, then looked down in her arms at the sleeping boy Joe. Her eyes filled with tears and her shoulders softened. She smiled and nodded. Compassion tempered with wisdom and a good dose of intelligence. "Thank you," She patted Jacob on the hand and closed her eyes.

Max had managed to pour his heart out to Denny before she left, telling her all about Clarissa and Jada. He was groveling with regret and apologies and practically begging her not to give up on him. It was more than she could take. The Hawaii trip was a godsend offering some breathing room and distance for her to work out all that she'd been through. Helen encouraged Denny to take the trip, offering to stay with Max and the kids to keep the bottom from falling out.

After the six-and-a-half-hour flight, they arrived at the Honolulu Airport and were greeted by two young vahine in long brightly colored dresses with bold tropical prints that are only appropriate on tropical islands. They welcomed Jacob, Jan, Lynn, Denny and little Joe with leis of fragrant plumeria blooms, warm smiles and ukulele tunes. The women were barefoot with slow moving hips and genuine smiles. The ride to the hotel was extended when Jacob realized the hotel he booked had no ocean view. He was on the phone rearranging and booking a different room, as they waited in the van. Denny thought the hotel was fine but didn't feel she was in a position to speak up. When they finally reached their rooms, she and Lynn settled in, and Jacob and Jan took a room a few doors down the hall. They were on the seventh floor of a condo style hotel, with sliding glass doors leading to a tight balcony overlooking Waikiki beach. The view was breathtaking. Emerald green and deep blue colors merged together with rolling whitecaps, breaking in the shallow waters along the shoreline. The beach was covered with rows and rows of rentable chaise lounges with cabanas of red, brown and bright turquois blue. Lynn plopped down on the bed next to little Joe, who was happily gurgling. "Why don't you go on and take a closer look," she suggested to Denny. "I think Joe would be fine for a little while. Go check out the beach."

"No," Denny protested. "I'm not gonna leave you here. We're in Hawaii! You have to come along." Lynn shrugged like she was indifferent.

"This is like my fifth or sixth trip. I'm fine. Go on. I'll watch Joe. Just don't be gone too long in case he gets worked up. I'm not real confident about comforting a newborn."

"I'll just run out and put my feet in for a few minutes, and then be back. We'll be going to dinner before long anyways, right?"

"Yeah. Go for it." Lynn returned to talking to Joe in a baby talk voice of googly gook, and was convinced she could make him smile, but he was only weeks old, and Denny chalked any smiles up to gas. She quickly ditched the socks and sneakers for flip flops, changed from her leggings to shorts, and grabbed the room key and was out the door. The beach was alive with activity. Suntanned teens with perfectly flat stomachs and carved bodies played volleyball, diving in the soft sand. A group of smaller kids dug deep water-filled moats for their sandcastles while their parents lay lazily nearby under the shelter of a beach umbrella. Body-boarding beginners in the shallow water played on the little breaking waves and others in deeper water sat on their surf boards waiting for the big ones. A wrinkly-skinned shell sleuth in a wide brimmed hat walked hunched over, carrying a little bucket and carefully examining the sand in front of her. Denny found an open space and stood looking at the water and listening to the surf. She was immediately comforted by the rhythm of the waves and warmth of the sun on her skin. She stood still and took it all in. *Be still and know that I am God.* Stillness was easy here. The occasional seagull called. The background noise of kids playing was muffled by the vastness of the beach and crashing waves. She closed her eyes. Waves. The edge of the ocean. Moving in and out. Endlessly. *What was it in Job, Lord? Waves that you set a boundary for. You may come this far and no more.* When Denny returned to the room, only twenty minutes later, Lynn was unpacking her suitcase into the armoire, "I claimed half of the dresser. I hope you don't mind. And we can get more hangers if we need to." Joe was sleeping where Denny had left him and she sat down to search for the scripture.

> *Who enclosed the sea behind doors*
> *when it burst forth from the womb,*
> *when I made the clouds its garment*
> *and thick darkness its blanket,*
> *when I fixed its boundaries*
> *and set in place its bars and doors,*
> *and I declared: 'You may come this far, but no farther.*
> *here your proud waves must stop'?*

"You look like you're on a mission," Lynn shut the door to the armoire and stuffed her suitcase in a corner near the bed that didn't contain little Joe.

"Oh," Denny said dreamily. "I was reminded of the story when God was lighting into Job like, 'Where were you when I created the sea and set its borders?' I had to find it. "Was everything okay with little Joe? Looks like he wasn't much trouble."

"Naw, he was fine. You could've stayed longer."

"I'm getting hungry! Any idea what the plan is?"

"If I know Jacob, he's gonna want to impress you. We're probably going to the Oceanarium. And don't ask. I'm not going to give it away, but you'll like it, I'm sure."

"I assume it's not casual, sandy feet in flip flops kind of thing?"

"Little black dress is probably more appropriate," Lynn chuckled. "Why don't you jump in the shower while Joe's still asleep, and I'll check with Jacob and Jan to see what the plan is."

The Oceanarium did not disappoint. One whole wall of the restaurant contained a three-story aquarium; 280,000 gallons of saltwater held in a 55x32 foot tank. The tank held sting rays, tropical fish, such as tangs, sturgeons and triggers. On the top near the surface were some big milkfish, some nearing five feet long. There was also a giant grouper and Great White Shark pup. Waiting for a table, Denny was surprised to see a scuba diver inside the tank. A mixture of prepared shrimp, squid and seaweed were hand fed to the fish allowing for up close examination for health issues. In the middle of the dining room was an enormous seafood buffet loaded with shrimp, scallops and clams cooked every which way. Steamed, fried and broiled to suit any fancy. Oysters and muscles surrounded huge fillets of mahi mahi, grouper, and piles of snow crab and king crab legs. A station in the middle offered prime rib with selected cuts and sizes carved by a jovial round Frenchman in a chef's hat. There were stainless steel pans of pasta, lobster casserole, creamed potatoes, corn casserole, macaroni and cheese, shrimp and crab casserole, all being replenished by the buffet staff with fresh pans of hot steaming crab legs catching Denny's eye each time they came from the kitchen. Little Joe snoozed quietly in his baby seat through the entire ordeal. Jan and Jacob and Lynn all took several trips to the buffet and the wait staff kept clearing the plates of crab leg shells as fast as they could fill them. Denny's eyes lingered over to the tropical fish peacefully showing off for the diners. After the third plate, she was slowing down, full and satisfied. Once or twice, she noticed Jacob seemed to be gazing at her. When Jan and Lynn took a trip to the restroom, he moved to be across from Denny. "I hope you like it," he said, a bit sheepishly.

"Are you kidding? It's amazing. What's not to like?"

He took his napkin and reached across the table to wipe a little butter from her chin. Normally she would have flinched at the proximity, but she had a little glow from the red wine and the rich food. She frowned slightly.

"Sorry. You had a little butter..er" Jan and Lynn returned and Denny put the gesture out of her mind, lifting Joe from his seat to go find a quiet place to nurse him. Back in the room, she and Lynn talked openly about Denny's life and circumstance, the baby Joe, the little girl Jada, the marital unrest. Lynn had troubles of her own. She was not your typical teenager. She seemed to Denny to be much older and more grounded than most. Lynn talked of her real father in the US. All of Jan's kids were raised in New York, and Jacob and Jan had only been together a few short years. Jan had mentioned how Jacob "saved her" and Denny didn't judge. They seemed very much in love, and it was obvious the kids loved him too. But Lynn, being the oldest had seen enough to know they were all better off.

The next day, Jacob rented a car and they took a drive to the Hanauma Bay Nature Preserve to do some snorkeling. The bay was breathtaking, and Denny was thrilled. Snorkeling was something she had always wanted to try, and her enthusiasm grew as they walked the long-paved path from the parking lot above to the beach below. The bay was shallow and rich with tropical color. Still waters of brilliant emerald, green, flecked with fall-like browns and oranges of living coral under the surface. The group had been instructed not to step on any coral and to float only. The sea turtles, fish and wildlife were to be observed but never touched or handled. The reef contained small lagoons and channels that led to the deeper waters of the outer reef. "We'll meet up at the car in two hours, in case we lose one another, which is very easy to do. In no time, the fish will have you in a different zone and it's easy to lose track of your surroundings when your eyes and ears are under water." Jacob settled into a beach chair under a couple of freakishly tall palm trees volunteering to keep little Joe protected from the sun while the rest swam. Denny stayed close to the rocky side of the reef and followed it along towards Witch's Brew. The water was calm and warm and shallow. She was enthralled by varying species of brightly colored fish. Schools of manini resembling tiny zebras darting to and fro. Powder blue tangs and emperor angel fish suited for a supermodel runway. The sights were overwhelming. The water began tossing her a bit as the waves picked up nearer the Witch's Brew. Denny lifted her head and discovered she had drifted quite further from shore than she intended. A wave crashed into the wall of rock beside her, splashing salt water into her face and mouth. She looked into the distance to see if she could see Jacob in his lawn chair, but the people were like twigs along the shoreline and another gust of water shoved her below the surface and into the rocks. Her snorkel filled when she tried to breathe and she choked and coughed her way to the surface. Pushing off the wall, she began the long swim to the beach, mask in one hand, and snorkel in the other. She felt foolish and reckless to have lost her bearings. She thought of her children back home, and her little Joe on the beach. What if he was awake and hungry? Would poor Jacob even know how to handle him? He was kind and grandfatherly, but did he even have children of his own? Her pace picked up, flipper clad feet moving firmly over the top of the water. When she finally reached the sand where the coral stretch along on each side, she stood up and looked around again. Her leg had a nasty gash in it that she hadn't noticed in the water.

"Trying to attract the sharks are ya?" Jen approached her from the beach and pointed to the bleeding gash in Denny's leg.

"Oh great," Denny moaned and hobbled over to the beach chairs where Jacob and Lynn were sitting. Little Joe slept in the shade underneath the back of Lynn's chair with a towel extended to a makeshift cabana. Denny sat in the sand and looked over her wound.

"Do we need to have it looked at? Stitches maybe?" Jacob sounded serious and concerned.

"It's a scratch, really. Just burns a little from the salt water," Denny said, grabbing a napkin from their picnic bag. She looked out over the bay, thankful to be safely back on shore. "Amazing. It's unbelievable how much beauty lies under that surface."

"Like another world," Jacob added.

"Yeah. I almost forgot about this one!" Denny laughed and Jan suggested they get back to the hotel and get ready for dinner. "Sushi tonight! And over dinner we can talk business about our work over here, and…" looking at Jacob, "we need to put Denny to work, and fill her in on the schedule. Would you mind watching the baby for a while after we eat?" She asked Lynn.

"Sure, that's why I'm here."

"Wait a second," Denny frowned, patting at her bleeding leg. "I thought I was here to keep Lynn company. I don't want her to feel like she has to be built-in childcare."

"Don't worry about it. I'm bored to death by all of their big plans. You go out and have a good time. And I can order in and watch Netflix and take care of little Joe. He's really a doll, Denny. Not exactly hard to care for. Anyways, he likes me. You see how he smiles at me."

"Uh hu. He's easy, I'll give you that, but those smiles…"

"Let her have her fantasies," Jacob interrupted. "It keeps her soft."

As the three of them left for dinner, Lynn was on the phone ordering room service. "Yes, I'll have the grouper sandwich with fries and the jalapeno basil slaw and a slice of key lime pie…no make that four slices of key lime pie…" Jan and Jacob were in the doorway enthusiastically giving the thumbs up.

"We love key lime. We'll all have some when we get back." Jan held the door as Denny kissed little Joe and grabbed her purse.

"We won't be late, hon." Denny added before she shut the door and followed them down the hall to the elevator.

Jacob was in the mood for a steakhouse, and the women did not object. Sushi tomorrow maybe. He was dressed in dark gray slacks with a belt that separated his two bellies. One above and one below. The pant legs were baggy with excess material. He looked like a man that may have lost a lot of weight, but still had fifty or more pounds to go. His jacket was large enough to button closed, which made the back and shoulders hang too loose. But he was neatly trimmed and shaven, his beard carefully manicured. His teeth white and clean. And he smelled good, a mixture of Irish Spring and Polo cologne. Jan wore a red and burgundy boho dress with a deep plunging halter top revealing generous cleavage. She wore her hair down and her sun-kissed skin glistened with fresh lotion and a hint of glitter. Her chunky heeled huarache sandals were woven in colorful leather. Jan had a bold, robust figure and a personality to match. She laughed loud. Shared her opinions freely, criticized without apology, and radiated confidence. Some people seem to be apologetic for their very existence, for taking up space on the planet. Jan was the opposite, donning an *I have every right to be here* attitude. Denny found her both refreshing and amusing.

The three of them were wolfing down buttered rolls and perfectly grilled steaks, loaded baked potatoes and a decent sized carafe of chianti. Jacob tried to explain his venture to Denny, but Jan interrupted him a number of times to keep him on topic. "He tends to ramble, giving you loads of useless and unnecessary information," she said at one point after bringing him back from the edge of oblivion.

"The thing is," continued Jacob, unhindered. "I am meeting with the mayor tomorrow. I have a proposal for him about a property on the island that could be utilized as a Bible college accreditation center. Bible colleges have no such entity to address the needs of colleges in the middle east, for example. There is no global organization. I intend to change that. What I need you to do, however, is research my ministry and name online and see what you come up with. I am concerned there are people trying to discredit me for their own gain. People who don't want to see a global accreditation organization."

"Okay…"

"Can you start tomorrow? I don't want you to work on it from you own computer, or from the hotel. I'd rather you find an internet café and take notes of all you find."

"Okay…" Denny was having a difficult time wrapping her head around this sort of work. It was not the *ministry* she had envisioned. But she decided she had a lot to learn, and maybe eventually it would lead to those tent meetings in Malawi. If she had any doubts, Jacob's extensive Bible knowledge and scope of pastoral experience kept her quiet.

Chapter 20

"Everything is fine here, honey. You just soak up some sun and enjoy your time away from the Yukon tundra! It's cold and dark here." Helen washed the breakfast dishes and thought of her daughter getting the first break from her life in years.

"I worry about Bishop and Alex. Are they doing okay?"

"Nothing to worry about. Bishop is her usual bouncy self, and Alex is very preoccupied with…"

"With Jada?" Denny guessed.

"Just don't you worry, honey. How's the baby? He nursing okay? And enjoying Hawaii?"

"He's great, Mom. I don't know if any baby has been this easy. Oh, maybe Amber. She hardly fussed a day in her life. But this little one just sleeps and eats and looks around with those huge brown eyes. He's so beautiful."

Helen didn't tell Denny about the adjustments around the house with Jada there. She was a lovely addition to the family, and immediately adopted by Alex, who thought a little Jamaican girl was the equivalent of a movie star, their deepest bond beginning when Jada had disappeared and Alex found her in the master bedroom, crying softly in her mom's bed.

"Hey," Alex snuck in quietly and sat beside her. "Hey little one. Whatcha doing?" She spoke gently and motherly. Jada looked up from her tear-soaked pillow.

"I miss my mom," she said between sobs and buried her face in the pillow again.

"Me too." Alex felt a lump in her throat thinking about her own mom and wished she were home already. Then she thought of poor Jada, whose mom would never come home. And she cried. Jada felt the bed shaking softly and lifted her eyes to see Alex hiding her face in her hands and she sat up, reached out and hugged her tight. They held each other like that crying softly in unison until Alex pulled away and looked at Jada's little face. Her skin was deep brown with eyes to match. She was an exotic new sibling with the darkest black shiny hair, thick wet eyelashes clumped together with tears. "Don't cry, Jada. Soon you'll have a mom again. And she won't be as beautiful and dark as yours, but you will love her."

Helen came in, finding the girls together and called them for dinner. She tussled their hair, first Alex, and then Jada, and led them to the table. Maxine and Helena were setting the table. Maxine was still bristly from her mother's mysterious dark baby, and sudden absence to "vacation" in Hawaii. Helena would pretend to be disgusted with the whole business, for Maxine's sake, but secretly had her own opinions. After all, Dad was home with this new addition from who knows where, and all of life seemed like one wild adventure in the Belanger house. Especially with Grampa Bishop coming and going. Everyone loved Bishop. He was such a novelty of a grandfather, famous and charismatic, gentle and handsome. They loved that he had been the one to bring Jada. And Jada treated him as if she'd known him forever and perhaps even better than any of them. There were currents of jealousy flowing throughout the family, but also, with Denny gone, a certain amount of grief and apprehension. None of the Belanger kids knew what the future held, and deep down, they were all scared by the shifting tectonic plates of their family. The uncertainty caused tension and irritability, but there were also moments of deep gratitude and honesty. Grandfatha was a rock to Jada. He promised to stay around until Denny returned. He stayed nearby, at the Hidden Valley Bed and Breakfast, but stopped in every day, often staying for dinner. Helen was grateful for the backup. Max had been home full time, but often hid himself away. He was not the boisterous Max the kids were used to. He was preoccupied, quiet, and somewhat mushy. The kids were not familiar with this side of their dad, and his morose nature caused them worry. Everyone was worried. Would anything ever be normal again?

The twins were off with friends a lot. It was easier to be out finding their way than home trying to figure out the puzzle their parents had created. They came in past curfew, and Helen gently talked with them about being careful and setting an example for Amber and Bishop..

"And Jada?" Maxine piped in with irritated sarcasm.

"Yes, Maxine. And Jada." Maxine sighed and went off to bed thinking she was the only sane one in the family. Helena grinned at her nana and shrugged and turned to follow Maxine to bed. "You could shift her opinion," Helen said to her second granddaughter. "She loves you very much, and she's hurting. I think she'd listen to you. We don't want her getting too carried away with bitterness and judgement."

Helena tilted her head to the side the way a golden retriever does when he's listening. She smiled and hugged her nana and thought about what she could say to soften her favorite twin sister. "I love you, Nana. I'm glad you're here. I sure wish mom would come back. I'd like to lay eyes on that baby brother of mine." Her eyes were glassy, and Helen pulled her close.

"It's all going to work out. I really believe that. And your mom will be home soon. Just work your magic on Maxine till she gets here, okay? Can you do that for me?"

Helena nodded and went off to bed. Bishop had gone, and Max had hidden himself away right after dinner. Jada and Bishop and Alex were all sleeping together in one room, giggling into the night. Helen thought of her Mark and gave him a call. He was beginning to wonder if she would ever return to Croghan.

"You know, I really think things will work out up here," she said to her sleepy husband. He laid in bed and cleared his throat. The three-hour time difference hadn't occurred to Helen until after he answered. "Oh gosh. I'm so sorry. It's nearly one in the morning there! I completely forgot."

"Don't worry about it. What's up? Obviously you are…still."

"Teenagers. Ugh," Helen sighed. "I'd forgotten how much work they are."

"Maybe you should come home and work on me," Mark still sounded sleepy. But at least he had a sense of humor.

"Maxine and Helena just got in, and I'm going to bed."

"When will you be back in my bed?"

"Soon I hope. Denny flies in on Friday, and if it all goes okay, I'll book a flight after a day or two."

"If it all goes okay?"

"Well, who knows. I may have to fly them all down and we'll have to help raise the kids, get the job done, you know."

"Yeah. I know," Mark sat up in bed and thought of Helen's huge heart toward Denny. "Helen don't get too tied up over it all. Denny's a smart girl, like her mother," Mark's voice was raspy with sleep. Helen thought it was sexy. Comforting. "Things will fall into place. Has Max fled the scene again?"

"No. Quite the opposite. Since his talk with Denny, he's been very serious and hasn't left the house. His father has been a big help to him, I think. And he keeps thanking me again and again for being here. Other than that, he's very quiet. I've never seen him like this." Helen sighed deeply and realized how tired she was.

"I miss you, Mark."

"Well, you should aim better next time."

"Funny man."

"I've been trying to tell you that for years. I love you, Helen. Get your cute curvy ass home."

"I love you, Mark. Soon I hope."

"Better be."

Chapter 21

Denny walked down the streets of Waikiki following the map to the cybercafé. The warm tropical air was like a soothing drug for her spirits. She was thankful and optimistic, holding her little baby bundle in a carrier on her chest. Along the sidewalks she passed several high-end jewelry stores and boutiques with name brand handbags and shoes that she'd never heard of and weaving between tourists and well-dressed professionals. She felt like an alien in a world of wealth. She and Max had never wanted for anything. Her home was grander than she ever needed, reliable cars, vans, and Jeeps over the years. Plenty of groceries and all she could ask for in maintaining a beautiful home. But her focus had been on educating and caring for the kids, exploring the wilderness of Canada, and homesteading skills like canning, baking, and gardening. She hadn't really browsed catalogs or magazines. She didn't know much about high-end fashion or brand names. She couldn't tell a Lamborghini from a Bentley. Just when she was beginning to feel like a frumpy housewife in a strange land, she ran smack into someone coming out the door of her destination. She had taken the thirty-minute walk from the hotel to Glazer's Café, crossing the Ala Wai canal and boathouse along Kapiolani Blvd to University Ave down South King Street to Glazers. She chose this route so she could stop in at an authentic dance supply store on the way back to the hotel.

The owner was friendly and helpful, albeit a little too chatty and self-aggrandizing for Denny's taste. He was about her age, maybe a little older. Thin, bald and not too bad to look at. He was trying to come off as laid back, but Denny thought he was high strung. Seemed to know a lot about everything. In a short span of time, he had gathered Denny was a born-again Christian on some sort of ministry errand. He was an easy conversationalist and confessed to be a basic run-of-the-mill hedonist. Denny wasn't entirely sure what a hedonist was. He gladly elaborated the simple philosophy of pleasure seeking as a way of life. He professed to being a millionaire a time or two. "Made it and lost it. Easy come, easy go. But now I've got this gig," he gestured to the large windows looking over the street. At first Denny assumed he was referring to owning the café, but soon he was expounding on another business entirely. "You see all those boutiques with Coach handbags and what not? I just send my girls out shopping. They come back with clearance items and I sell them to the Japanese on eBay. You should try it!" He enthusiastically walked Denny over to a closet, opened the door and declared, "My office and shipping room!" The closet was filled with flattened boxes and mailing tape and shipping labels. "All I do is sit here and list them and watch the money roll in."

"Interesting," Denny felt she was getting an education wherever she turned. She had a little experience with eBay. But nothing on this scale. Plus, she didn't live in Hawaii, so access to discounted brand names wasn't very feasible.

"Let me get you set up," the hedonist was saying, as he pulled out a chair in front of a computer. "What exactly are you looking for? Do you need any help?"

He's friendly enough, Denny thought. Certainly not a threat. "I'm trying to see what's out there in cyber land on my boss, er, pastor, friend." He made a face like he understood. Denny wasn't sure she did. But before she knew it, there were little tidbits of information on Jacob Netto and the world-wide ministry he headed. Denny made notes of all the web addresses, the content, the good, the bad, and the ugly. Every now and then Mr. Hedonite would wander over and look over her shoulder to ask how she was doing.

"Interesting," she said. And kept on jotting down notes. When she finished up, she went to the lounge area of the café, where college kids sat and drank cappuccinos and lattes. She ordered a decaf and sat in a discreet corner to nurse little Joe, who had been happily napping, attached to her in his carrier as usual. The coffee tasted great. Had it been earlier in the day, she would have ordered the real thing, but it was close to two pm, and caffeine after two never ended well. When she had strapped Joe into his pouch again, she grabbed her notes and headed back toward the hotel. The dance shop on her way had a full selection of hula supplies. A wall of multicolored Tahitian Hau skirts, made from thick rafa, woven lauhala mats, Samoan jewelry, ceremonial headdresses, and fire knife practice batons and lovely Tahitian prints and sarongs. The place was filled with an island feel, barefoot sales attendants and Hawaiian Reggae music that Denny couldn't help but move to. She thought of the Shakira video Hips Don't Lie, and her teens laughing in the living room trying belly dance moves in front of the TV. Her heart ached to have them all here. Maxine and Helena would love this store, Amber would be doting over Joe and happy just to be with her mama. She was a mommy's girl for sure. Alex would have been thrilled with the seafood buffet and the aquarium and Jacob and Jan, always thrilled to be with new people. Bishop was her water lover from birth and would have been in heaven in Hanauma Bay snorkeling and exploring the vast array of fish varieties. Denny sighed and thought of Max. And this new Jada. It troubled her to think of them. She was not a part of that club. It was a part of Max's world that she didn't want to know about. But there was no avoiding it anymore. Denny had left for Hawaii before Bishop brought the child around. She didn't feel strong enough to be around for the introductions. Helen encouraged her to go off with little Joe and focus on her own feelings for a change. She was well able to step in and fill the gap. And she was quite firm about it. Denny felt lost and vulnerable and did as her mother suggested. *Sometimes you don't trust your own judgement. In those times, it's good to rely on the people you know love you most.*

On the last night in the hotel, after dinner, Jan called the room. "What's going on? Joe asleep?"

"As usual," Denny chuckled, "Why?"

"Come on down here for a minute. I want to ask you about something." Denny walked the three doors to Jacob and Jen's room and Jan let her in. "Jacob went down to grab a snack. You want a glass of wine?"

"Sure," Denny took the champagne flute and sipped the dry Chardonnay. Jan was looking at her as if she had a confession. Denny waited.

"You like Jacob, don't you?"

"Of course."

"Well. You like him like *that?*" Jan was watching her again as though some big revelation was about to unfold.

"Not sure what you're getting at, Jan." Denny frowned.

"Look. He's a great man. And his one unfulfilled fantasy is to be with two women at once. I can't believe he's never done it! I just want to make that happen for him."

Denny sat stunned and swallowed hard so she wouldn't spit her wine all over the place.

"Oh come on. Don't act so shocked. Surely it's not a big deal for you. You're no prude."

"Um," Denny stuttered. "I really don't know what to say. But no. No thank you. That won't be happening." Suddenly Jan's face turned red. She was getting impatient.

"Are you kidding me? No?" she huffed and continued, "Why do you think we brought you here?"

Denny's head was spinning. She set down her glass and walked toward the door. Jacob passed her in the doorway, asking, "You alright?" He seemed sincere enough. Denny walked past him and back to her room. Lynn was watching tv and talking on her phone. Little Joe was lying on the bed cooing happily. She went into the bathroom, stripped down and took a long, long shower, the words *stupid! stupid! stupid! Naïve idiot!* going over and over in her mind as she scrubbed her skin till it hurt.

Chapter 22

Things were quiet in the airport. Conversation was spotty at best. Jacob kept asking if anything was wrong. Denny eyed a kiosk filled with freshly made leis. She went and purchased one and approached Jacob as he sat on the wide wooden slat bench. "Thank you for this trip, Jacob," she said quietly as she put the lei over his head and whispered in his ear, "and this is the only 'lei' you'll get from me." His eyes grew wide and he looked shocked.

"Is that what you think this is about?" Denny ignored his protest and walked away. She retrieved little Joe from Lynn's arms and stayed with her the rest of the trip. Lynn seemed the most sane of the three, and she appreciated her company. On the long flight home, she kept thinking how stupid she was. Ironically, Jacob's words came to her, "Try treating yourself like you are helping one of your children." She shook her head and thought of her children. She couldn't wait to get home, even with the ground shaking beneath it. She missed her kids terribly and didn't like experiencing so much without them. Looking over the trip, most of it was enchanting and some of it was eye opening. The things she had discovered on the internet about Jacob and his ministry concerned her, but she had been giving him the benefit of the doubt. Surely he couldn't be a con man to people in faraway poverty-stricken countries. Charging hundreds of dollars for some membership certificates, only to leave them dry and full of empty promises. There were pending lawsuits and angry victims scattered among the stories she read. But the man she knew spoke eloquently at Passover dinners and loved Jan's children and could listen for hours with compassionate skill and interest way beyond the best shrink or therapist. He was a gentle giant. Was he a liar? A fraud? Denny didn't know what to think. Eventually she relied on her go to method of coping…*Be thankful. Find the good.* It was a beautiful getaway (until the last night). A wonderful experience. Joe had been a peach. Lynn was solid. And they'd always have Passover. Poor Alex. She thought of her love for the Netto family, Jacob, Jan and all the kids. She'd be heartbroken. Denny would have to think of creative ways to avoid them, and hope Alex would be distracted by other things. Jada. Yes, I'm sure Jada will keep her mind occupied for a while. And Bishop too, if he's sticking around.

Denny rested her head against the window and tried not to be anxious. She tried to remember the sound of the ocean that had calmed her to the core. *Please, Lord. Let me keep some of that calm. I'm yours. You guide my steps. The way you contain the ocean and keep it from flooding the whole earth. The way you say, "this far and no more".*

Be my walls and boundaries. My life feels like turbulent waters. An ocean of upheaval. You are my hiding place. My sea anchor. Save us, Lord. And we will be saved.

Chapter 23

Bishop and Helen sat at the kitchen island in the wee morning hours whispering about Max and Denny and the mess they were in, sipping coffee and ceasing conversation when the teens appeared. Maxine and Helena grabbed some granola bars, Mountain Dew, yogurt, and a zip lock bag of fresh fruit and stuffed it into backpacks. "How about a sandwich, girls? I can make you some tuna salad, or there's cold meat?"

"Thanks Nana, this is good." The girls kissed Nana and then Bishop. Helena abruptly stopped and turned on the way out, "Will you be here this afternoon, Grampa?" Bishop smiled and nodded, deciding he certainly would. The kids were lovely and he enjoyed them so much that he had made arrangements with a realtor to buy a home in Whitehorse. He could stay there for the short summers, and travel to his other home in Texas when the cold weather became unbearable. He also noticed the sprawling cabin was a little neglected. He could stick around and help Max with needed repairs. Max was used to being on the road and had a lot of work to do if he was going to be at home more. He barely noticed the home needed new roofing, a few window replacements, a fresh stain on the logs, and more winterizing to keep the drafts out. In the meantime, Bishop hoped to get him some help. He was obviously depressed and overwhelmed. He couldn't continue hiding out in the bedroom, barely eating, sleeping for hours on end, the only sound from the space was the occasional flushing of the toilet. He had come to dinner most nights, and tried to muster up some life, some of the old Max that the kids knew and loved. But it was all he could do to just not cry, let alone be the life of the party. Bishop and Helen talked it over and tagged teamed him when the kids weren't around.

"We think you need to get some help. Preferably before Denny comes home. We're worried about you. I've called around and found a good psychiatrist. And I'll drive you myself." His dad was gentle, but firm. Helen stood by nodding sympathetically. Max looked at his dad with a blank expression.

"I can drive. Where is it?" Max reached out for the papers his dad was holding. "Can't hurt," he mumbled and shuffled away to the bedroom, returned a few minutes later wearing a clean shirt, grabbed his keys, and kissed a worried looking Helen on the forehead. "Thank you. Both of you. For all you've done." He started to get choked up as he made his way to the door. "Hope they take walk-ins." He shut the door behind him and Helen and Bishop looked at each other shaking their heads.

"Doubtful. But maybe they'll take a look at him and admit him!"

"Oh, Lord. I hope they don't COMmit him!" Helen joked. Only she wasn't really joking. Max returned later in the day with a couple of prescriptions and a book about bipolar disorder. Helen made a big pot of penne pasta with a creamy vodka sauce. The kids tidied up the house, tiny Bishop picked up all the toys and clutter and put them where they belonged. Amber and Alex swept and vacuumed, Jada insisted on helping and said she knew how to clean an entire apartment by herself. So Helen gave her a cloth and some dusting spray and set her free. The tile floors were mopped and dishes done. The house smelled of lemon Pledge and warm garlic bread. Max showered and shaved and looked almost like his old self, except in the eyes, which were far away and empty. He cleaned out the wall sized stone fireplace in the family room and built a good roaring wood fire. The girls came in excitedly from class shouting, "Look what we found fresh from the tropics!"

Denny and the girls had hugged and cried in the driveway, Helena snatching little Joe from Denny's arms and cooing over him as they went inside. Maxine grabbed Denny's luggage and looked her over. "Quite the tan you have there, world traveler!" Denny squeezed Maxine again and whispered, "I missed you so much."

Inside, the table was set for eleven. Bishop, Helen, Max, Denny, Maxine, Helena, Amber, tiny Bishop, Jada and Little Joe, who even had a highchair pulled up to the table to set his carrier seat on. Joe was being passed around and ogled by Helen and Bishop. Amber managed to get to her mother and hug her tight. She teared up at the sight of her. Denny felt like she should sit on the couch so everyone could have a piece of her and take turns getting all the love. She was about to make her way over when she caught a glimpse of some very dark hair around the corner. Huge brown eyes were looking warily at Denny. Jada was taking in the scene of all the kids mauling their mama. When Denny's eyes met hers, the rest of them followed her gaze and got quiet. For a moment, everyone was aware of poor Jada's predicament. Denny said quietly, "Why don't you all have a seat at the table for a minute? I'll join you after I meet this little one."

Jada backed away shyly and Denny noticed Max across the room watching her. The silence was deafening. Moments passed with nothing but the crackling fire in the other room. Finally, Bishop rose and walked to Jada, squatting down behind her. He began to speak quietly, looking over her shoulder at Denny, "Well, well. Looks like another big day for you, hu sweetie? Jada turned and hugged her grandfatha and buried her face in his sweater.

"You've been so very brave, Jada. So very strong. I'm sure your mama is proud of you. Looking down from heaven. You're gonna be okay. Remember? Everything's gonna be okay." He rubbed her hair softly and

Denny stood watching. It was all she could do not to sob. She looked back at Max, who was also trying hard not to lose it, and around the table full of kids holding their breath. Helen held Joe who never made a peep. Bishop wiped Jada's face with his handkerchief, stood up and extended a hand for her to hold. She took his hand and he walked her past Denny to her seat at the table. Jada's eyes went back and forth from Denny to Max.

"Garlic bread! Shit," Helen handed little Joe to Amber breaking the spell everyone was under and ran for the oven.

"Nana swore!" little Bishop covered her mouth with her hand. Max and Denny's eyes met and they both smiled. Then they started laughing. They walked quickly toward each other and embraced, holding the hug for a long time. Jada got down from her seat at the table and shyly moved toward Denny. She tugged at her shirt, and Denny looked down. The biggest brownest eyes she'd ever seen were smiling at her. She bent down and shook her little hand. "It's nice to meet you, Jada. Do you like hugs?" Jada nodded and wrapped her arms around Denny's neck. Denny pulled her little brown body close to hers, noticing her skin color was only a shade lighter than little Joe's. She looked up at Max and shook her head at the irony of it all. Max was still glassy eyed and smiling.

Chapter 24

Lynn was nearly screaming on the other end of the line. Denny struggled to understand her. "Honey, slower. Speak slower. I don't know what you're saying."

"The house is on fire!"

"Oh my God. Are you safe? Where are you?"

"We're outside! The fire trucks are here…Jacob and Jan went to Juneau!"

"I'll be right there. Everyone is safe?"

"Yes, we're okay." She sounded a little calmer but Denny rushed to the river home. The Netto kids were huddled together in the yard and the house was in flames. She hurried them into the vehicle and left, so they didn't have to watch it burn to the ground. All the girls were sobbing. Lynn sat in the back seat with arms around Ally and Kyle and Jess. They were all in nightgowns and tee shirts and sleep shorts and were shivering to the bone. Denny brought them in and told them to get by the fire. Helena put on a kettle for cocoa and Alex started going through the cupboards making a snack plate for them. Triscuits, Tortilla chips, club crackers, cheese, pepperoni, olives. Amber pulled out a loaf of bread and made sandwiches, while Helena sat with them in the living room, offering blankets and dry clothes. After a while they settled down and Denny got the story. Ally was quick to blame Kyle and Jess for playing with a candle. It somehow caught the bedroom curtain on fire and the flames went crazy. There was no stopping it. They called 911 and ran outside while the blaze grew brighter. After a brief talk with a firefighter, they were left alone standing there and watching with horror. That's when they called Denny. They were getting worked up and hysterical again talking about it so Denny hushed them and quieted them and told them they were safe. Drink up. Helena was holding out mugs of cocoa. Denny got a call just as they were settling down again.

"Is this Denny Belanger?" The voice was harsh and authoritative.

"Yes. Who's calling?"

"Ma'am, this is Officer Maddock with the Royal Canadian Mounted Police. Do you have the children of Jan Velia in custody from their riverfront home?"

"Yes. They called me less than an hour ago as their house was burning down."

"Ma'am, you need to bring them to us immediately," Denny thought he clearly misunderstood the kids' predicament.

"Bring them where?" She asked with some confusion.

"To the home. Where they called from."

"The house that is in flames? No. I can't do that. These kids are very shaken up, and I've barely gotten them to settle down. And you want me to bring them back there?"

"Yes ma'am. And immediately."

"No," Denny was shaking now. There's no way these kids should be taken back to that scene. And with Jacob and Jan out of town, she was the only comfort they had at the moment. "If you want them, you can send someone to come get them. I cannot bring them back there." She hung up the phone and paced the kitchen. She knew they would be on their way to retrieve the kids and the time was short. When flashing lights appeared in the driveway, they all began crying again. Lynn tried to be the rock and quiet them, while Denny grabbed warm clothes from the closet. Winter coats, boots, scarves, hats, mittens. "Here," Denny said, "put these on, quickly. You're gonna be fine. I promise. Just bundle up and go with the policeman. No one's going to hurt you. You're safe. You didn't do anything wrong," Denny followed them out to the car and handed them the box of Triscuits, hollering as they drove away, "Everything's going to be okay."

Later that night they got a call from a distraught Jacob. He was making no sense on the phone but was on his way over. Max and Denny put the kids to bed. Enough excitement for one day. They put on a pot of coffee and waited for Jacob. Twenty minutes later a very distraught Jacob was at the door. "Can I use your computer? Please?"

He was out of breath, and already walking toward the corner of the living room where he'd seen Denny or one of the kids using it. He sat with his wet boots, hunched over the screen waiting, waiting. Dial up. Ugh. Flecks of snow were still in his white hair, his hands red from the cold.

"You want some coffee, Jacob?" Denny asked. He didn't answer. She turned to Max. He shrugged. They both waited. After a while Jacob began to ramble, without looking up from the computer. He was nearly panicked. Blurting things out.

"Jan's in jail. I've got to get her out of there."

"Jail?" Denny and Max said in unison.

"Parental abduction."

"Hu?"

"She missed a custody hearing with her ex. Technically HE has custody of them. And when the fire and rescue came, along with the police, they ran her name and as soon as we arrived from Juneau, the Mounties were there to pick her up. The kids are on their way to the states to be delivered to their father." Denny and Max stood stunned. Jacob was a mess. He looked like he would break down crying at any moment, but then would shift into paranoid ramblings about the fire. "They're after me. I mean. I can't even access my accounts. They've been frozen." Suddenly he sprang up out of his chair and looked desperately at Max. "Can I borrow some cash? Please. I can't let her stay in a jail cell. Will you go with me? I just need a thousand for bail money. And as soon as I get my accounts straightened out, I'll reimburse you. Please." The way he said please was more of a command than a plea. He wasn't begging. He was desperately depending on us doing the right thing. Max went to the office and retrieved cash from the safe, grabbed his keys and shrugged at Denny, who was at a loss for what to do.

"See you…when you get back. I guess." And they were out the door. The men returned with Jan an hour or so later. She was her usual boisterous self. Talking and laughing out loud about the adventures of getting arrested. She was clearly wound up and Denny didn't know if she was putting on a show, trying to hide her fear or if she really was having a good time. "It was just like the book of Acts, I tell ya! I talked to all the other women about Jesus and salvation. It was wild!"

No mention of the kids. Denny didn't bring it up. She did notice, however from some paperwork left on the island in the kitchen that Jan's last name was not Netto at all. It was Velia. Janice Adoloratta Velia. Denny gathered that she was still married to her ex-husband. And she and Jacob were doubtfully married at all. The guest bedroom was made up for them. Regardless of what was true or untrue about them, they had both experienced a great deal of upheaval and were exhausted. Denny was doubtful that Jacob would settle down, but retrieving Jan seemed to help bring him from the edge. When they had gone to bed, Max sat on a barstool in the kitchen.

"He says they'll be moving on. Wants me to pick up the reigns of his ministry work. A worldwide network of small independent churches."

"Uh hu. I don't know. I think there's a lot of angry parishioners out there."

"Maybe we could make a difference." Max looked strangely hopeful. Denny watched him, trying to figure out what he was thinking. Never a good idea. But this was the first time in twenty years of marriage that Max had expressed an interest in anything Bible related. Denny was quiet. She allowed herself to imagine Max in Jacob's shoes. Going to help ministers around the globe with their missions. Max had a big heart, and who was she to say whether or not God was calling him in some way. Still. Her experiences with Jacob and Jan and their work made her doubtful. But there were those pictures. Photos of Jacob in Malawi, surrounded by young church leaders and children. The mailings she had done to Pakistan, membership certificates to dozens of churches, around the world. But there were also the emails. The angry ones who wanted their money back. "You did nothing for us! You did not do what you promised!" By the next morning, Denny had envisioned a network of people and churches around the world that she and Max could interact with. Find out what they need. Jump in. We can be the change. Perhaps we can get money FOR them! We can host fundraisers. We live in one of the wealthiest countries in the world. We can share our knowledge, travel and get involved personally. Still. There were doubts.

Jacob and Jan were on the road and headed for Alaska first thing in the morning. Still no mention of the kids or their father, but it was clear she wasn't going to fight it out in court. They were on the run. Max and Jacob shook hands and when the door shut behind their unusual guests they looked at one another and shook their heads. *Wow.*

A few days passed and the police were at their door again. "Subpoena", the man said handing Denny an envelope. "You've been served," and he turned and walked away. Max appeared from stoking the fire.

"What was that?"

"Subpoena?"

"What?"

Denny shrugged and opened the envelope with Max looking on. "It appears to be a summons to court. You, Max Belanger, the *new president* of the World Church Alliance are being sued for fraud!"

"What the…" Max took the paper from Denny and read it through. "Oh shit." They spent the next couple of hours on the computer. They looked over the WCA website which belonged to Jacob. There was an announcement on the home page declaring Max Belanger the new President of WCA and all correspondence could be directed to him, as Jacob Netto would be stepping down for a sabbatical, the time frame of his return undetermined. The emails poured in until Max had to change his address. Fortunately, when he explained to the judge the circumstances of his association with Jacob Netto and Jan Velia, how he'd bailed her out of jail and they left town the next day. How he had no clear picture of what the "ministry" was. The judge shook his head and dismissed the case.

"We're only out a thousand dollars," he said to Denny when he got home.

"Well, they did pay my way in Hawaii."

"Eh," Max shook his head and they were both quiet.

"What a ride," he said after a while, grinning.

Chapter 25

Maxine and Helena completed their associate degrees in Yukon. Helena had decided to pursue nursing and Maxine comparative literature. But their greatest interest was the Emerald Coast in Florida. They fantasized about endless beaches of white sand and turquoise water. "It's your fault, Mom," Maxine joked with Denny. "All those pictures from Hawaii, the aquarium, the surfers. We never had an inkling to go beach bound before that."

When Denny had returned from her Hawaii trip she gathered everyone in the living room and made them get comfortable while she put on some tropical hula music. She made virgin piña coladas, coring the pineapple, mixing it with coconut cream, coconut milk and lime and served them in the pineapple topped with maraschino cherries. She disappeared again after delivering the drinks and returned wearing a heavy grass skirt that sat on her hips with a wide belt woven with little white shells and tropical halter top covered with bright red and orange hibiscus flowers. Her arms were loaded with leis which she placed on the head of each of her children kissing them on the cheek. "Aloha, and Mahalo. She stepped back and began to move to the music, putting on a little luau performance. As she danced she said, "Mahalo means thank you. And I'm so thankful for all of you. Thank you for parting with me for a time. It was very helpful, and I hope I can bring just a little bit of paradise back to you." She passed out gifts she had collected on her trip, a book of sea life for little Bishop, a signed CD from a renown Hawaiian ukulele player for Alex. For Amber, bracelets made from tiny seashells, each string a different kind, all stacked in a row. For Maxine and Helena, she had collected a dozen aloe, coconut, and honey facial masks to do a spa day, along with some delightful coconut lotion that smelled like the Hawaiian tropics. Jada sat wide eyed staring a Denny. Her eyes followed as she distributed gifts and her heart was wild with anticipation. But she was also filled with a dread that there would be no gift for her. She was dark as night compared to these half siblings. And though Denny had been kind and warm to her, she thought it just a matter of time before they all sent her away. Maybe to Jamaica, the faraway land her mother had told her about. A place of sundresses and dark skin and beautiful braids. Where brilliant flowers and wildly colorful birds were everywhere. Nothing like Chicago, her mother told her. No snow. No skyscrapers. Just palm trees and sunshine.

Denny looked at Jada and smiled. She had saved her gift for last. She reached into the bag and pulled out four strands of lei kukui nut beads, two black and two white. She took a white strand and combined it with a black strand and draped them over Jada's neck, kissing her on the cheek. Then placed the other set of one black and one white over Max's neck, kissing him on the cheek. Denny had decided in the dance supply store the day she saw the beads that she would stay with Max and she would take in Jada. She didn't really feel she had a choice, but being away in Hawaii, she could pretend it was her decision. In her heart, she knew all along she would take care of Max's child. And Max. Jada hopped off the couch and went from Alex to Maxine to Helena to Amber and Bishop, eventually standing over little Joe in his seat showing her beads with great pride. "Aren't they beautiful? And look! Black ones too! Just like you and me." She dangled the black beads over little Joe. The girls watched her enthusiasm and enjoyed her immensely. Maxine grabbed her from behind, wrapped her arms around her waist and hoisted her onto her lap. She burrowed her face into Jada's neck and smiled, looking at Max, and then her mom. She felt a glimmer of hope that her family may not be that absurd after all.

Gulf Coast State college in Panama City Florida sounded like a dream world to Maxine and Helena. They had never been out of Canada and were ready to launch.

"Just let me know when you're arriving and I'll fetch you from the airport. You *have to* stay with me!" Melissa was beside herself. She and Denny had talked periodically over the years, but Denny was so grounded with her large family, that Mel only saw her if she took the trip to Canada. And Melissa was no fan of the cold dark weather up there. She had come after Maxine was born, and again after Helena, waiting until the babies were old enough to at least hold their head up and do something other than cry and poop. Melissa showered them with gifts and attention and enjoyed the time with Denny. She was very happy Denny had found her soul mate and seemed genuinely content with her budding family. But it wasn't Melissa's cup of tea. And she didn't hang around too long.

"Come on a getaway with me. I'll fly you to Bermuda and we can drink Mimosas and talk about the good times."

"These are good times."

"Yeah. They are. But I miss you. I wish you lived closer. You'd love Florida." Melissa had bought a condo on the ocean overlooking the gulf coast. She pestered Denny several times to come visit, but then gave up, as Denny was always either pregnant or nursing a baby. When she finally called saying her kids wanted to check out the college, Melissa dropped the phone in excitement. "Wait! Wait!" she hollered as she retrieved the phone after kicking it under the table. Finally, out of breath and lying on the floor she panted, "Wait! Hello? Are you still there Denny?" She heard a chuckle from Denny and continued, "Oh my God! Did you say the kids want to come to Gulf Coast College?" That's like five minutes from me! Oh God, they'll love it here. I can be like their God mother and look out for them."

"I'm counting on it. Max and I are going to fly down with them and take a look around."

"You have to stay with me. I have an awesome three story with an elevator. You can have the guest suite. It's on the ground floor with a deck right on the beach. There's a master bedroom and bath and another guest bedroom upstairs the girls can share. Oh, I can't wait. When are you coming? I'll pick you up."

"No, Mel. Don't worry about that. Max and I will rent a car and come to you after we tour the college. We promised the girls we could stay a couple days, but not long, because we're not bringing the rest of the kids. Max's dad, Bishop volunteered to keep them at his house while we're away. Of course they were thrilled."

"I would be too! How is that old fox doing? Damn he's good looking."

"Getting older Melissa. Like we all are! I can't wait to see you! I'll fill you in with the details soon!"

"I'm so excited, Denny! It's been too long. You just made my day."

"I know. Me too! I can't wait to see you."

Max's arms were around her from behind as she hung up the phone. "You realize she's the reason we're together?"

"Of course," Denny jerked her head as he tickled her neck with bristly kisses. He hadn't shaved in a few days. She wanted him to grow out a short beard to see how he looked.

"You were in total denial. Pretending you would never marry. Didn't want kids. Didn't remember ever saying you did…"

"Psh. Nonsense."

Jada was pushing a two-year-old Joe in a stroller around the twists and turns of the heated tile floors. She grabbed his sippy cup off the counter and dumped its contents in the sink, rinsed it out and went to the fridge for milk. "You want milk or water Joe Joe? You can't have more juice, you've had enough." He smiled a huge gurgley smile and his eyes lit up at the milk as she screwed the top on and handed it to her little brother. The two brown-skinned, brown-eyed kids disappeared around the corner as Max and Denny looked on. When their eyes met, they smiled, their hearts full of the wonder of it all.

Max raised an eyebrow. "We're a kid shy of your declaration. You said eight."

"Yeah. That was before I experienced teenagers. I think seven is plenty."

Bishop walked in the door with a big smile and an armload of groceries.

"What you got there?" Max said, shutting the door behind him.

"Steaks, crab legs, shrimp, scallops and all the fixings for loaded baked potatoes and a salad. We're celebrating!"

"What are we celebrating?" Max said, unloading the goods onto the counter as Denny watched. Jada, Joe, Amber, Alex and Bishop all came running when they heard Bishop come in.

Bishop spoke with a mysterious hush to his voice, and his eyes were dancing. "We landed the mother lode, Max. A contract for the Smithsonian."

"You're kidding me. We got it?"

"We got it."

"The National Museum of Indigenous Peoples of the World" Bishop spoke the words slowly and over Denny and all the kids as if her were a priest speaking a blessing over them. In a way, he was. The project would secure their financial freedom for life.

"Does this mean we will move to America?" Alex was always itching for exciting news. She was hoping the Smithsonian was in Los Angeles.

"I just bought a house here, Alex. You can't go moving away. Besides," Bishop said, "you and the rest of these monsters are coming to my house next week, remember? An overnight adventure for a few days. It will have to hold you over till you're old enough to move to Hollywood." Alex's wheels turned, thinking about the Smithsonian, Hollywood, and then resting on the idea of a few days at Bishop's. Then she smiled. Yes. A few days with a famous grandfather would certainly do. She stuffed her hand in one of the grocery bags and pulled out a live lobster. "Woah!" She swung it around lunging its spindly moving legs at Jada and little Bishop, who was now a nine-year-old bean pole, almost the same height as Alex. She shrieked out loud as Alex laughed. Jada stared at the creature wide eyed, and Joe's little head went from Alex, to Bishop, to Jada. Alex slowly crouched down and used her boogie man voice, taking steps toward little Joe in his stroller. "Whooo will eat whooo for dinner?" As she got closer to little Joe, Denny piped up,

"Careful Alex. Those little legs still have pincers, even if the big ones are rubber banded." Alex frowned, looked skeptical and examined the lobster closer.

"Eww" she tossed the whole thing in the sink. "You're right!"

"Of course I'm right. I'm the mom." Denny started pulling out the big steamer pots and the stainless salad bowl, unpacking and unwrapping food, moving around on autopilot while watching Max and his father discuss timelines and plans.

The Smithsonian, she repeated to herself, impressed. The Smithsonian. Wow.

All characters appearing in this work are fictitious. Any resemblance to real persons, living or dead, is completely coincidental.

ALSO BY MARY JOSLYN

JOURNEY OF LIFE SERIES
Blood Soaked Earth
The Cottage
Roskilde
Harvest

OTHER BOOKS
The Greatest Gift